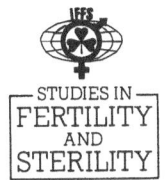

STUDIES IN
FERTILITY
AND
STERILITY

The
Male Factor
in
Human Infertility
Diagnosis
and
Treatment

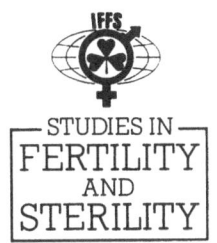

STUDIES IN
FERTILITY
AND
STERILITY

The
Male Factor
in
Human Infertility
Diagnosis
and
Treatment

Edited by
W. Thompson, R.F. Harrison
and J. Bonnar

Themes from the XIth World Congress on Fertility and Sterility,
Dublin, June 1983, held under the Auspices of the International
Federation of Fertility Societies

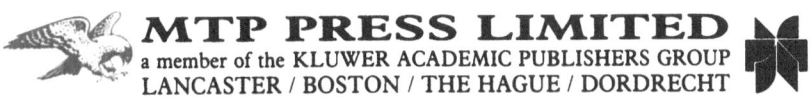

MTP PRESS LIMITED
a member of the KLUWER ACADEMIC PUBLISHERS GROUP
LANCASTER / BOSTON / THE HAGUE / DORDRECHT

Published in the UK and Europe by
MTP Press Limited
Falcon House
Lancaster, England

British Library Cataloguing in Publication Data

World Congress on Fertility and Sterility
(11th : 1983 : Dublin)
The male factor in human infertility diagnosis and treatment.—
(Studies in fertility and sterility)
1. Infertility, Male
I. Title   II. Thompson, William, *1937*–
III. Harrison, R.F.   IV. Bonnar, J.
VI. International Federation of Fertility
Societies   VI. Series
616.6'92   RC889
ISBN-13: 978-94-010-8669-1   e-ISBN-13: 978-94-009-4898-3
DOI: 10.1007/978-94-009-4898-3

Published in the USA by
MTP Press
A division of Kluwer Boston Inc
190 Old Derby Street
Hingham, MA 02043, USA

Library of Congress Cataloging in Publication Data

Main entry under title:

The male factor in human infertility diagnosis and management.

(Studies in fertility and sterility)
Includes bibliographies and index.
1. Infertility, Male—Congresses. 2. Artificial insemination,
Human—Congresses. I. Thompson, W. II. Harrison, R. F.
(Robert Frederick) III. Bonnar, John. IV. International Federation
of Fertility Societies. V. World Congress on Fertility and Sterility
(11th : 1983 : Dublin, Dublin) VI. Series. [DNLM: 1. Infertility,
Male—diagnosis—congresses. 2. Infertility,
Male—therapy—congresses. 3. Insemination,
Artificial—congresses. WJ 709 M244 1983]
RC889.M33   1984   616.6'92   84-21321

Phototypesetting by
Georgia Origination, Liverpool

Contents

Preface   xi

List of Contributors   xiii

Section 1: Evaluation of the spermatozoa

1   A computerized technique for the measurement of sperm cell velocity: correlation of the results with *in vitro* fertilization assays
W. V. Holt, H. D. M. Moore, A. Parry and S. Hillier   3

2   Automatic analysis of sperm characteristics by means of a micro-computer system
M. Hazama, H. Okada, O. Matsumoto, S. Kamidono and J. Ishigami   9

3   *In vitro* cross penetration testing in infertile couples
U. Braun, T. Katzorke and D. Propping   13

4   A new standardized *in vitro* penetration test (bovine) measuring the capacity of fertilization. I
G. Corradi, G. Gimes, I. Süle and F. Balogh   17

5   A new standardized *in vitro* penetration test (bovine) measuring the capacity of fertilization. II
G. Gimes, G. Corradi and F. Balogh   23

6   Penetration of zona-free hamster eggs by human spermatoza. Comparison of two methods
M. Gelas, E. Warembourg, B. Sele, C. Osto Rero, C. Estrade and P. Jalbert   27

7   Reduced penetration of zona-free hamster ova by cryopreserved human spermatozoa
D. Navot, E. J. Margalioth, N. Laufer and J. G. Schenker   33

8   Effect of caffeine on human sperm penetration into zona-free hamster ova
    E. J. Margalioth, D. Navot, J. Y. May, N. Laufer, J. Ovadia and J. G. Schenker   37

9   The variability and clinical value of a heterologous ovum penetration test
    P. L. Matson, J. P. Pryor, R. Curson and W. P. Collins   41

10 Laser-induced stimulation of sperm motility *in vitro*
    H. Sato, M. Landthaler, D. Haina and W.-B. Schill   47

11 Time-sequential observation on human sperm penetration into zona pellucida-free hamster oocytes by scanning electron microscopy
    M. Suzuki, A. Tsuiki, K. Hoshi, K. Kyono, H. Imaizumi and H. Hoshiai   51

12 Analysis of various experimental conditions on the rate of human sperm penetration into zona-free hamster ova
    E. J. Margalioth, D. Navot, R. Rabinowitz, N. Laufer, R. Voss and J. G. Schenker   57

Section 2 The Biochemistry of Gonadal Function

13 Levels of vitamin B_{12} and folic acid in seminal plasma from subjects with normal semen analysis and patients with idiopathic oligoasthenozoospermia
    M. Brassesco, A. Oliver, R. Moreno, F. Morer and R. Vila   63

14 Functional role of relaxin in human seminal fluid
    F. Krassnigg, E. Töpfer-Petersen, J. Frick and W.-B. Schill   69

15 Hyperprolactinaemia and abnormal seminal cytology
    D. Sultan Sheriff   73

16 Serum FSH and spermatogenesis
    J. H. Nelson, III, C. B. Paschall, III, W. Baird, R. C. Harsh and M. A. Davis   79

17 Response to FSH of human Sertoli cells in culture
    V. Santiemma, N. Casasanta, P. Rosati, S. Moscardelli, G. Iapadre and A. Fabbrini   85

18 Anaerobic urinary and prostatic bacteria, and prostatic biochemical markers in urine after prostatic massage of infertile men
    P. J. Moberg, P. Eneroth, J. Lizana and C. E. Nord   91

19 Effects of bombesin on the pituitary response to TRH and LHRH in humans
    C. Scarpignato, G. Baio and A. E. Pontiroli   95

CONTENTS

Section 3 Immunology and Male Reproduction

20 Characteristics of a monoclonal anti-human sperm antibody
    L. Mettler, V. Baukloh and S. Paul   101

21 Topographical analysis of the surface of human spermatozoa by means
    of monoclonal antibodies
    A. C. Hinrichsen, M. J. Hinrichsen and W. -B. Schill   105

22 Human seminal plasma proteins: identification and preliminary
    characterization of a human sperm coating antigen (h-SCA) protein in
    physiological and pathological conditions
    G. Lombardi, M. De Rosa, L. Quagliozzi, M. Minozzi, P. Abrescia, J.
    Guardiola and S. Metafora   111

23 Antigenicity of sperm cells after freezing and thawing
    M. Phillip, D. Kleinman, G. Potashnik and V. Insler   117

24 A radioimmunoassay for antisperm antibodies using ^{125}I-labelled
    protein A
    D. Cannon, G. McKenna, J. Harney, J. Barron, B. M. Coughlan and D.
    Powell   123

25 Human cervical response to artificial insemination
    I. J. Pandya and J. Cohen   127

Section 4 Medical Treatment of the Infertile Male

26 Kallman's syndrome – sustained spermatogenesis three years after
    cessation of treatment
    A. I. Traub, A. B. Atkinson and W. Thompson   135

27 Effects of testosterone undecanoate on semen quality and sexual
    behaviour
    D. Da Rugna and J. Saastamoinen   139

28 Tamoxifen in the treatment of reduced semen quality: preliminary
    results
    E. W. Jecht, C. Hirschhäuser and W. Krause   143

29 Tamoxifen in the management of male subfertility – a retrospective
    analysis
    G. Lunglmayr, U. Maier and Ch. Kratzik   147

30 Increased sperm count in 41 cases of idiopathic normogonadotropic
    oligozoospermia following treatment with tamoxifen
    J. Buval, K. Ardaems-Boulier, A. Lemaire, J. C. Fourlinnie and M.
    Buvat-Herbaut   151

31 Treatment of oligozoospermia with Chinese herb medicine
    H. Yoshida, Y. Naitoh, M. Watanabe and K. Imamura   155

32 Bacterial contamination of semen of infertile couples and the effect of antibiotic treatment of semen quality and fertility
M. Shilon, Y. Stadtmauer, M. Holzinger, B. Bartoov and C. Bahary 161

Section 5 Surgical Treatment of the Infertile Male

33 Effects on semen parameters and pregnancy rate after occlusion of the spermatic vein in subfertile men with idiopathic varicocele
U. Maier, G. Lunglmayr, P. Riedl and W. Kumpan 169

34 Varicocelectomy for oligozoospermia
N. Anandan, R. C. L. Feneley and J. C. Gingell 175

35 Emission failure due to retroperitoneal lymphadenectomy: first report of a pregnancy after insemination of spermatozoa obtained by midodrin-induced retrograde ejaculation
W. -B. Schill and W. Bollamnn 181

36 Restoration of antegrade ejaculation following radical retroperitoneal lymphadenectomy
D. Kröpfl, M. Meyer-Schwickerath, G. Plewa, R. -H. Ringert and R. Hartung 187

37 Transurethral resection of verumontanum for ejaculatory duct stenosis and oligozoospermia
C. C. Carson 191

38 Results of microsurgical testicular autotransplantation in nine patients with high-lying undescended testis
H. Garibyan, F. W. J. Hazebroek, J. C. Molenaar and N. F. Dabhoiwala 197

Section 6 Artificial Insemination

39 Echosonographic control of follicular growth in heterologous therapeutic insemination (AID)
V. Ruiz-Velasco, O. B. de la Pena, E. D. Domville and E. M. Zelaya 205

40 A comparison of fresh and frozen semen in AID practice
W. H. Bleichrodt and H. G. Mutke 209

41 AID in the problem patient
T. Karzorke and D. Propping 217

42 Repeat pregnancies with AID
B. N. Barwin 223

43 The post-insemination test in predicting the outcome of artificial insemination with husband's semen
S. Friedman 227

CONTENTS

44 The relationship between the survival of human spermatozoa in culture medium and pregnancy rate
    H. Key and S. Avery   233

45 Duration of vitality and migrating ability of +4 °C cryopreserved human spermatozoa
    E. Kesserü and C. Carrere   237

46 Male sterility caused by anejaculation – aetiology diagnosis and treatment
    Z. Zuckerman, Y. Tadir and J. Ovadia   243

47 Psychological patterns of AID-demanding marital couples
    *O. Todarello, F. M. Boscia, G. A. Patella, M. W. La Pesa, F. Matarrese,
    L. Natilla and A. Taranto*   247

48 The complexity of psychological issues involved in artificial insemination by donor
    R. Rowland   257

49 Secrecy in the provision of artificial insemination by donor (AID)
    R. Snowden   261

Addendum to Section 1

50 Relationships between results of post-coital test and parameters of semen analysis
    G. B. La Sala, L. Dessanti, A. M. S. Foscolu, G. Ghirardini and F. Valli   265

Addendum to Section 2

51 Seminal plasma isoenzyme LDH-X values in extreme oligozoospermia
    P. Cvitković, M. Gavella, Z. Papić, Z. Singer and Z. Škrabalo   271

    Index   275

Preface

This book is a compilation of edited papers which were presented at the XIth World Congress of Fertility and Sterility held in June 1983 in Dublin, Ireland. Although it has long been known that male factors are responsible in at least 30% of infertile couples only recently have concerted efforts been made on the part of urologists, gynaecologists and basic scientists to identify these factors more precisely.

The nature of spermatogenesis is complex but application of various scientific methods have at last opened up new and promising approaches to our understanding of this subject. Clinical results however have been depressing; the majority of treatments lack realistic evaluation and are initiated in hope rather than with a sound scientific basis. We anticipate that this volume will in some small way correct these deficiencies.

The papers have been grouped into related topics. The first section deals with the evaluation of the spermatozoa and includes a critical assessment of the recently introduced zona-free hamster egg test of sperm function. Further sections include the biochemistry of gonadal function and the immunology of male reproduction; most papers are concerned with studies in the human. The clinical sections cover medical and surgical approaches to treatment and the final section deals with various aspects of AID practice.

To each of the authors we express our sincere thanks for their contributions in providing subject matter which reflects the state of the art' in so many important areas. We also express our gratitude for the unfailing help we received from the staff of MTP Press in the preparation of this volume.

William Thompson
Robert F. Harrison
John Bonnar

Ireland, September 1984

List of Contributors

P. ABRESCIA
Institute of General Physiology
Faculty of Sciences, University of Naples
via Mezzocannone 8
I-80100 Naples
ITALY

N. ANADAN
Department of Surgery
Glan Clwyd Hospital
Bodalwydan, Rhyl
Clwyd LL18 5UJ
UNITED KINGDOM

K. ARDAENS-BOULIER
Service d'Endocrinologie USNA
Avenue du Pr Laguesse
F-59037 Lille
FRANCE

A. B. ATKINSON
Metabolic Unit
Royal Victoria Hospital
Belfast BT12 6BA
UNITED KINGDOM

J. AVERY
Dr B A Mason's Clinic
25 Weymouth Street
London W1N 3FJ
UNITED KINGDOM

C. BAHARY
Department of Gynecology and Obstetrics
Meir Hospital, Sapir Medical Center
Kfar Saba
ISRAEL

G. BAIO
Department of Biomedical Sciences
University of Milan
S. Raffaele Hospital
I-20100 Milan
ITALY

W. BAIRD
Department of Obstetrics and Gynecology
St Anthony Hospital
1450 Hawthorne Ave
Columbus, OH 43203
USA

F. BALOGH
Department of Obstetrics and Gynecology
Semmelweis University Medical School
Budapest
HUNGARY

J. BARRON
Department of Immunology
Mater Hospital
Eccles Street
Dublin 7
IRELAND

B. BARTOOV
Department of Life Sciences
Bar-Ilan University
Ramat-Gan
ISRAEL 52100

B. N. BARWIN
Department of Gynecology/Infertility
770 Broadville Ave, Suite B-1
Ottawa, Óntario K2A 3Z3
CANADA

xiii

V. BAUKLOH
Department of Obstetrics and Gynecology
University of Kiel
Hegewichstrasse 4
D-2300 Kiel 1
WEST GERMANY

W.-H. BLEICHRODT
Praxis für Fertilitäts-störungen und
  Instrumentelle Inseminationen
Winterthurerstrasse 5
D-8000 Munich 71
WEST GERMANY

W. BOLLMANN
Department of Obstetrics and Gynecology
Klinikum Grosshadern
University of Munich
Marchioinistrasse 15
D-8000 Munich 70
WEST GERMANY

F. BOSCIA
Clinica Ostetrica e Ginecologica
Università degli studi di Bari
Corso Vittorio Emanuele II, 48
I-70100 Bari
ITALY

M. BRASSESCO
Servicio de Laboratorio
Fundación Puigvert
Cartagena No. 340
Barcelona 25
SPAIN

U. BRAUN
Fertility Institute
Kettwiger Strasse 2–10
43 Essen 1
WEST GERMANY

J. BUVAT
Association pour l'Etude de la Pathologie de
  l'Appareil Reproducteur
49 rue de la Bassée
F-59000 Lille
FRANCE

M. BUVAT-HERBAUT
Association pour l'Etude de la Pathologie de
  l'Appareil Reproducteur
49 rue de la Bassée
F-59000 Lille
FRANCE

O. BUZO DE LA PENA
Centro Para El Estudio de la Fertilidad
Temistocles 210
Mexico City
11560 MEXICO

D. E. B. CANNON
Department of Endocrinology
Mater Hospital
Eccles Street
Dublin 7, IRELAND

C. CARRERE
Department of Reproduction
I. Cátedra de Ginecología
Av. Córdoba 2331
(1120) Buenos Aires
ARGENTINA

C. C. CARSON
Division of Urology
Duke University Medical Center
Durham, NC 27710, USA

N. CASASANTA
Department of Medical Sciences
School of Medicine, University of l'Aquila
V. le Duca degli Abruzzi 3/A
I-67100 l'Aquila
ITALY

J. COHEN
Department of Zoology and Comparative
  Physiology
University of Birmingham
Birmingham B15 2TT
UNITED KINGDOM

W. P. COLLINS
Department of Obstetrics and Gynaecology
Kings College Hospital
Denmark Hill
London SE5 8RX
UNITED KINGDOM

G. CORRADI
Department of Obstetrics and Gynecology
Semmelweiss University Medical School
Budapest
HUNGARY

B. M. COUGHLAN
Department of Gynaecology
Mater Hospital
Eccles Street
Dublin 7, IRELAND

LIST OF CONTRIBUTORS

R. CURSON
Department of Obstetrics and Gynaecology
Kings College Hospital
Denmark Hill
London SE5 8RX
UNITED KINGDOM

P. CVITKOVIĆ
Vuc Vrhovac Institute
Krijesnice bb
4100 Zagreb
YUGOSLAVIA

N. F. DABHOIWALA
Department of Urology
Academic Medical Centre of Amsterdam
Meigbergdreef 9
1105 AZ Amsterdam Zuid-Oost
THE NETHERLANDS

D. DA RUGNA
Universitäts Frauenklinik
CH-4031 Basel
SWITZERLAND

M. A. DAVIS
Department of Pathology
St Anthony Hospital
1450 Hawthorne Ave
Columbus, OH 43203, USA

M. DE ROSA
Department of Endocrinology
2nd School of Medicine
University of Naples
Via S Pansini 5
I-80100 Naples
ITALY

L. DESSANTI
Division of Obstetrics and Gynecology
Santa Maria Nuova Hospital
I-42100 Reggio Emilia
ITALY

E. DOMVILLE
Centro Para El Estudio de la Fertilidad
Temistocles 210
Mexico City
11560 MEXICO

P. ENEROTH
Research and Development Laboratory
Department of Obstetrics and Gynecology
Karolinksa Sjukhuset
S-104 01 Stockholm, SWEDEN

C. ESTRADE
Laboratoire Biologie de la Reproduction
Faculté de Médecine
Grenoble
FRANCE

A. FABBRINI
Department of Medical Sciences
School of Medicine, University of l'Aquila
V. le Duca degli Abruzzi 3/A
I-67100 L'Aquila
ITALY

R. C. L. FENELEY
Department of Urology
Southmead Hospital
Westbury on Trym
Bristol BS10 5NB
UNITED KINGDOM

S. A. M. FOSCOLU
Division of Obstetrics and Gynecology
"Francini" Hospital
Montecchio Emilia
Reggio Emilia
ITALY

J.-C. FOURLINNIE
Association pour l'Etude de la Pathologie de
l'Appareil Reproducteur
49 rue de la Bassée
F-59000 Lille
FRANCE

J. FRICK
Department of Urology
Landeskrankenanstalten Salzburg
Salzburg, AUSTRIA

S. FRIEDMAN
Tyler Medical Clinic
921 Westwood Boulevard
Los Angeles CA 90024, USA

H. GARIBYAN
Department of Urology
Academic Medical Centre of Amsterdam
Meibergdreef 9
1105 AZ Amsterdam Zuid-Oost
THE NETHERLANDS

M. GELAS
Laboratoire Biologie de la Reproduction
Faculté de Médecine
Grenoble
FRANCE

G. GHIRARDINI
Division of Obstetrics and Gynecology
"Franchini" Hospital
Montecchio Emilia
Reggio Emilia
ITALY

G. GIMES
Department of Obstetrics and Gynecology
Semmelweiss University Medical School
Budapest
HUNGARY

J. C. GINGELL
Department of Urology
Southmead Hospital
Westbury on Trym
Bristol BS10 5NB
UNITED KINGDOM

J. GUARDIOLA
CNR International Institute of Genetics and
  Biophysics
via Marconi 10
I-80125 Naples
ITALY

D. HARIMA
Radiation and Environmental Research
  Center Munich
Ingolstädler Landstrasse 11
D-8042 Neuherberg
WEST GERMANY

J. HARNEY
Department of Endocrinology
Mater Hospital
Eccles Street
Dublin 7
IRELAND

R. C. HARSH
Department of Pathology
St Anthony Hospital
1450 Hawthorne Ave
Columbus, OH 43203
USA

R. HARTUNG
Department of Urology
University of Essen
D-4300 Essen
WEST GERMANY

M. HAZAMA
Department of Urology
Kobe University School of Medicine
5-1 Kusuoki-cho 7-chome
Chuo-ku, Kobe 650
JAPAN

F. J. W. HAZEBROOK
Department of Paediatric Surgery
Sophia Kinderziekenhuis
Gordelweg 160
3038 GE Rotterdam
THE NETHERLANDS

A. C. HINRICHSEN
Department of Obstetrics and Gynaecology
University of Munich
Maistrasse 11
D-8000 Munich 2
WEST GERMANY

M. HINRICHSEN
Department of Obstetrics and Gynaecology
University of Munich
Maistrasse 11
D-8000 Munich
WEST GERMANY

H. C. HIRSCHHÄUSER
Department of Urology
St Josephkrankenhaus
Walderstrasse 34–38
D-4010 Hilden
WEST GERMANY

W. V. HOLT
Gamete Biology Unit
Department of Reproduction
The Zoological Society of London
Institute of Zoology
Regent's Park
London NW1 4RY
UNITED KINGDOM

M. HOLZINGER
Department of Gynecology B
Meir Hospital, Sapir Medical Center
Kfar Saba
ISRAEL

K. HOSHI
Department of Obstetrics and Gynaecology
Sendai Shakaihoken Hospital
16–1, Tsutsumi-machi 3-chome
Sendai 980
JAPAN

LIST OF CONTRIBUTORS

H. HOSHIAI
Department of Obstetrics and Gynaecology
Sendai Shakaihoken Hospital
16-1, Tsutsumi-machi 3-chome
Sendai 980
JAPAN

G. IAPADRE
Department of Medical Sciences
School of Medicine, University of L'Aquila
V. le Duca degli Abruzzi 3/A
I-67100 L'Aquila
ITALY

H. IMAIZUMI
Department of Obstetrics and Gynaecology
Tohoku University School of Medicine
1-1 Seiryo-machi
Sendai 980
JAPAN

K. IMAMURA
Department of Urology
Showa University
1-5-8 Hatanodai, Shingawa-ku
Tokyo 142
JAPAN

V. INSLER
Department of Obstetrics and Gynecology
Soroka Medical Center
PO Box 151
Beer Sheba 84 101
ISRAEL

J. ISHIGAMI
Department of Urology
Kobe University School of Medicine
5-1 Kusunoki-cho 7 chome
Chuo-ku, Kobe 650
JAPAN

P. JALBERT
Laboratoire Biologie de la Reproduction
Faculté de Médecine
Grenoble
FRANCE

E. W. JECHT
Department of Dermatology
University of Erlangen, School of Medicine
Hartmannstrasse 14
D-8520 Erlangen
WEST GERMANY

S. KAMIDONO
Department of Urology
Kobe University School of Medicine
5-1 Kusunoki-cho 7 chome
Chuo-ku Kobe 650
JAPAN

T. KATZORKE
Fertility Institute
Kettwiger Strasse 2-10
D-4300 Essen
WEST GERMANY

E. KESSERU
Department of Reproduction
I. Cátedra de Ginecología
Av. COordoba 2351
(1120) Buenos Aires
ARGENTINA

H. KEY
Dr B A Mason's Clinic
25 Weymouth Street
London W1N 3FJ
UNITED KINGDOM

D. KLEINMAN
Department of Obstetrics and Gynecology
Soroka Medical Center
PO Box 151, Beer Sheba 84 101
ISRAEL

F. KRASSNIGG
Department of Dermatology, Andrology Unit
University of Munich
Frauenlobstrasse 9-11
D-8000 Munich 2
WEST GERMANY

Ch. KRATZIK
Departments of Obstetrics and Gynecology 1
University of Vienna Medical School
Vienna, AUSTRIA

W. KRAUSE
Department of Dermatology
University of Marburg
Deutscherrnstrasse 9
D-3550 Marburg
WEST GERMANY

D. KROPFL
Department of Urology
University of Essen
Huffeland Strasse 55
D-4300 Essen
WEST GERMANY

W. KUMPAN
Department of Radiology
University of Vienna Medical School
Alserstrasse 4
A-1000 Vienna, AUSTRIA

K. KYONO
Department of Obstetrics and Gynaecology
Tohoku University School of Medicine
1–1 Seiryo-machi
Sendai 980, JAPAN

M. LANDTHALER
Department of Dermatology
Frauenlobstrasse 9–11
D-8000 Munich 2
WEST GERMANY

W. M. LA PESA
Clinica Psichiatrica II
Università degli studi di Bari
Corso Sonnino 54/b
I-70121 Bari
ITALY

G. B. LA SALA
Division of Obstetrics and Gynecology
Santa Maria Nuova Hospital
I-42100 Reggio Emilia
ITALY

N. LAUFER
Department of Obstetrics and Gynecology
Hadassah University Hospital
POB 12000 Jerusalem 91120
ISRAEL

J. LIZANA
Pharmacia Fine Chemicals
S-751 04 Uppsala
SWEDEN

A. LEMAIRE
Association pour l'Etude de la Pathologie de
l'Appareil Reproducteur
49 rue de la Bassée
F-59000 Lille
FRANCE

G. LOMBARDI
Department of Endocrinology
2nd School of Medicine
University of Naples
via S. Pansini 5
I-80100 Naples
ITALY

G. LUNGLMAYR
Urologische Universitätsklinik Allgemeines
Krankenhaus
Alserstrasse 4
A-1090 Vienna, AUSTRIA

U. MAIER
Department of Urology
University of Vienna Medical School
Alserstrasse 4
A-1090 Vienna, AUSTRIA

E. J. MARGALIOTH
Department of Obstetrics and Gynecology
Hadassah University Hospital
POB 12000 Jerusalem 91120
ISRAEL

F. MATARRESE
Clinica Psichiatrica II
Università degli studi di Bari
Via Principe Amedeo 334
I-70100 Bari
ITALY

P. L. MATSON
Department of Obstetrics and Gynaecology
Kings College Hospital
Denmark Hill, London SE5 8RX
UNITED KINGDOM

O. MATSUMOTO
Department of Urology
Kobe University School of Medicine
5–1 Kusunoki-cho 7 chome
Chuo-ku, Kobe 650
JAPAN

J. Y. MAY
Obstetrics and Gynecology Department
Beilinson Medical Center
Tel Aviv
ISRAEL

M. MAYER-SCHWICKERATH
Department of Urology, University of Essen
Hufeland Strasse 55
D-4300 Essen
WEST GERMANY

G. McKENNA
Department of Endocrinology
Mater Hospital
Eccles Street
Dublin 7
IRELAND

LIST OF CONTRIBUTORS

S. METAFORA
CNR Institute of Molecular Embryology
via Toiano 2
80072 Arco Felica
Naples
ITALY

L. METTLER
Department of Obstetrics, Gynecology and
  Reproductive Biology
University of Kiel
Hegewichstrasse 4
D-2300 Kiel
WEST GERMANY

M. MINOZZI (deceased)
Department of Endocrinology
2nd School of Medicine,
University of Naples
via S. Pansini 5
80100 Naples
ITALY

P. J. MOBERG
Department of Obstetrics and Gynecology
Södersjukhuset
S-100 64 Stockholm
SWEDEN

J. C. MOLENAAR
Department of Paediatric Surgery
Sophia Kinderziekenhuis
Gordelweg 160
3038 GE Rotterdam
THE NETHERLANDS

R. MORENO
Department of Hematology
Fundacion Puigvert
Barcelona
SPAIN

F. MORER
Servicio de Andrología
Fundación Puigvert
Cartagena No. 340
Barcelona 25
SPAIN

S. MOSCARDELLI
Department of Medical Sciences
School of Medicine, University of L'Aquila
V. le Duca degli Abruzzi 3/A
I-67100 L'Aquila
ITALY

H.-G. MUTKE
Praxis für Fertilitätsstörungen und
  Instrumentelle Inseminationen
Drygalskiallee 117
D-8000 Munich 71
WEST GERMANY

Y. NAITOH
Department of Urology
Showa University
Y-S-8 Hatanodai
Shinagawa-Ku
Tokyo 142
JAPAN

L. NATILLA
Clinica Psichiatrica II
Università degli studi di Bari
Via S.L. Filippini II
I-70032 Bitonto (BA)
ITALY

D. NAVOT
Department of Obstetrics and Gynecology
Hadassah University Hospital
POB 12000 Jerusalem 91120
ISRAEL

J. H. NELSON
Department of Urology
St Anthony Hospital
1450 Hawthorne Avenue
Columbus, OH 43203
USA

C. E. NORD
Karolinska Institutet
National Bacteriological Laboratory
S-105221 Stockholm
SWEDEN

H. OKADA
Department of Urology
Kobe University School of Medicine
5-1 Kusunoki cho 7-chome
Chuo-Ku, Kobe 650
JAPAN

A. OLIVER
Servicio de Laboratorio
Fundación Puigvert
Cartagena No. 340
Barcelona 25
SPAIN

C. OSTORERO
Laboratoire Biologie de la Reproduction
Faculté de Médecine
Grenoble
FRANCE

J. OVADIA
Department of Obstetrics and Gynecology
Beilinson Medical Center,
University of Tel Aviv Medical School
Petah Tikva 49100
ISRAEL

I. J. PANDYA
Department of Obstetrics and Gynecology
University of Birmingham
Birmingham Maternity Hospital
Edgbaston
Birmingham B15 2TG
UNITED KINGDOM

C. B. PASCHALL
Department of Obstetrics and Gynecology
St Anthony Hospital
1450 Hawthorne Avenue
Columbus, OH 43203
USA

G. PATELLA
Clinica Psichiatrica II
Università degli studi di Bari
Via Fosse ardeatine 42
I-70023 Gioia del Colle (BA)
ITALY

S. PAUL
Department of Obstetrics and Gynecology
University of Kiel
Hegewichistrasse 4
D-2300 Kiel 1
WEST GERMANY

M. PHILLIP
Department of Obstetrics and Gynecology
Soroka Medical Centre
PO Box 151
Beer Sheba 84 101
ISRAEL

G. PLEVIA
Department of Dermatology
University of Essen
Hufeland Strasse 55
D-4300 Essen
WEST GERMANY

A. PONTIROLI
Department of Biomedical Sciences
University of Milan
S. Raffaele Hospital
I-20100 Milan
ITALY

G. POTASHNIK
Department of Obstetrics and Gynecology
Soroka Medical Center
PO Box 151
Beer Sheba 84 101
ISRAEL

D. POWELL
Department of Endocrinology
Mater Hospital
Eccles Street
Dublin 7
IRELAND

D. PROPPING
Fertility Institute
Keltwiger Strasse 2–10
D-4300 Essen 1
WEST GERMANY

J. PRYOR
Department of Urology
Kings College Hospital
Denmark Hill
London SE5 8RX
UNITED KINGDOM

L. QUAGLIOZZI
Department of Endocrinology
2nd School of Medicine
University of Naples
Via S. Pansini, 5
I-80100 Naples
ITALY

R. RABINOWITZ
Department of Obstetrics and Gynecology
Hadassah University Hospital
POB 12000 Jerusalem 91120
ISRAEL

P. RIEDEL
Department of Radiology
University of Vienna Medical School
Alsterstrasse 4
A-1000 Vienna
AUSTRIA

LIST OF CONTRIBUTORS

R. H. RINNGERT
Department of Urology
University of Essen
Hufeland Strasse 55
D-4300 Essen
WEST GERMANY

P. ROSATI
Department of Medical Sciences
School of Medicine, University of l'Aquila
V. le Duca degli Abruzzi 3/A
I-67100 L'Aquila
ITALY

R. ROWLAND
Lecturer in Social Psychology Humanities
Deakin University
Humanities, Deakin University
Victoria 3217
AUSTRALIA

R. VELASCO
Cemtro Para El Estudio De La Fertilidad
Temistocles 210
Mexico City 11560
MEXICO

V. SANTIEMMA
Department of Medical Sciences
School of Medicine, University of L'Aquila
V. le Duca degli Abruzzi 3/A
I-67100 L'Aquila
ITALY

H. SATO
Department of Dermatology
Andrology Unit
Frauenlobstrasse S-11
D-8000 Munich
WEST GERMANY

C. SCARPIGNATO
Laboratory of Clinical Pharmacology
Institute of Pharmacology
University of Parma
I-43100 Parma
ITALY

J. G. SCHENKER
Department of Obstetrics and Gynecology
Hadassah University Hospital
POB 12000
Jerusalem 91120
ISRAEL

W. B. SCHILL
Department of Dermatology
Andrology Unit
University of Munich
Frauenlobstrasse 9-11
D-8000 Munich
WEST GERMANY

B. SELE
Laboratoire Biologie de la Reproduction
Faculté de Médecine
Grenoble
FRANCE

DR. M. SHILON
Department of Gynecology B
Meir Hospital Sapir Medical Center
Kfar Saba 44 Abiwa St
Ra'anana 43263
ISRAEL

R. SNOWDEN
Institute of Population Studies
University of Exeter
Hoopern House
101 Pennsylvania Road
Exeter EX4 6DT
UNITED KINGDOM

J. STADTMAKER
Department of Gynecology B
Meir Hospital, Sapir Medical Center
Kfar Saba
ISRAEL

I. SULE
Department of Obstetrics and Gynecology
Semmelweiss University Medical School
Budapest
HUNGARY

D. SULTAN-SHERIFF
Department of Biochemistry
Faculty of Medicine
University of Garyounis
PB 1451
Benghazi
LIBYA

M. SUZUKI
Department of Obstetrics and Gynecology
Tohoku University School of Medicine
1-1 Seiryo-machi
Sendai 980
JAPAN

Y. TADIR
Infertility Clinic
Department of Obstetrics and Gynecology
Beilinson Medical Center
University of Tel Aviv Medical School
Petah Tikva 49100
ISRAEL

A. TARANTO
Clinica Psichiatrica II
Università degli studi di Bari
Viale O. Flacco, 47/a
70100 Bari
ITALY

W. THOMPSON
Department of Midwifery and Gynecology
Queen's University Belfast
Belfast BT7 1NN
NORTHERN IRELAND

O. TODARELLO
Clinica Psichiatrica II
Università degli studi di Bari
Via Papa Innocenzo XII 66
70124 Bari
ITALY

E. TOPFER-PETERSON
Department of Dermatology Andrology Unit
University of Munich
Frauenlobstrasse 98–11
D-8000 Munich 2WG
WEST GERMANY

A. I. TRAUB
Department of Midwifery and Gynecology
Queen's University Belfast
Belfast BT7 1NN
NORTHERN IRELAND

A. TSUIKI
Department of Obstetrics and Gynaecology
Tohoku University School of Medicine
1-1 Seiryo-machi
Sendai 980
JAPAN

F. VALLI
Division of Obstetrics and Gynecology
Santa Maria Nuova Hospital
42100 Reggio Emilia
ITALY

R. VILA
Servicio de Laboratorio
Fundación Puigvert
Cartagena No. 340
barcelona 25
SPAIN

R. VOSS
Human Genetics Department
Hadassah University Hospital
POB 12000
Jerusalem 91120
ISRAEL

E. WAREMBOURG
Laboratoire Biologie de la Reproduction
Faculté de Médecine
Grenoble
FRANCE

M. WATANABE
Department of Urology
Showa University
1-5-8 Hatarodai
Shiragawa-Ku
Tokyo 142
JAPAN

H. YOSHIDA
Department of Urology
Showa University
1-5-8 Hatanodai
Shinagawa-Ku
Tokyo 142
JAPAN

E. M. ZELAYA
Centro Para El Estudio de la Fertilidend
Temistocles 210
Mexico City
11560
MEXICO

Z. ZUCKERMAN
Infertility Clinic
Department of Obstetrics and Gynecology
Beilinson Medical Center
University of Tel Aviv Medical School
Petah Tikva 49100
ISRAEL

Section 1

Evaluation
of the
Spermatozoa

1
A computerized technique for the measurement of sperm cell velocity: correlation of the results with *in vitro* fertilization assays

W. V. HOLT, H. D. M. MOORE, A. PARRY and S. HILLIER

INTRODUCTION

Amongst the parameters available for study in the clinical investigation of human male fertility by semen analysis, the quantitative determination of sperm motility is possibly one of the most useful, although it is also one of the most demanding measurements to perform. Subjective scoring systems for the assessment of motility[1] have, therefore, been used extensively in experimental and diagnostic work, whilst the precise measurement of sperm velocity or of wave motions in a semen sample has mainly been confined to the research laboratory.

In this paper a rapidly performed but accurate method for measuring sperm velocity is described which would be suitable for use in a routine clinical laboratory. In an effort to test the diagnostic value of velocity measurements, a correlative study is described here in which the predictive value of mean velocity is examined in relation to success in the zona-free hamster oocyte sperm penetration assay. This assay is regarded, in this context, as a good indicator of male fertility[2].

MATERIALS AND METHODS

Fifty-five semen samples were used in this study. They were obtained from the

3

husbands of women attending an *in vitro* fertilization clinic. Initially there was no reason to suppose that these men were subfertile.

Velocity measurements on undiluted semen were performed within 4 hours of collection, and the first sperm dilution procedure for the sperm–ovum interaction assay was carried out within 1½ hours of collection. The techniques used in performing the zona-free hamster egg penetration assay have been described previously[3,4].

Velocity measurements were performed using a semi-automatic image analysis system (VIDS, Micromeasurements Ltd., UK) which comprised an Apple computer and graphics tablet linked to a television camera. This was in turn mounted upon a Zeiss standard microscope equipped with a ×40 phase contrast objective and heated stage (30 °C).

For examination, $20 \mu l$ of undiluted semen was mounted beneath a 22×22 mm glass coverslip, giving a depth of $41 \mu m$. The image of the moving spermatozoa was displayed on the TV monitor together with a mobile cursor, controllable via the graphics tablet. Using computer graphics a grid of 2×5 rectangles was also displayed as an aid to sampling.

Measurement of sperm velocity was achieved by tracking the chosen spermatozoon with the cursor, using the graphics tablet and pen to control cursor movement. The track of each spermatozoon was displayed as a series of points, ten such points being plotted per second. Using the co-ordinates of each point the total distance travelled was computed, which together with the time taken to the nearest 0.1 s yielded the mean velocity for each cell.

In this study, 50–60 spermatozoa from each semen sample were measured in this way. In an effort to randomize the selection of spermatozoa, cells were selected as they entered each of the ten rectangles in turn. They were then tracked over distances of 100–200 μm; the computer was programmed to reject measurements if they were completed in less than 1 s. This condition usually applied only when spermatozoa were moving especially fast.

RESULTS AND DISCUSSION

The method described here for the measurement of sperm velocity was simple to perform and required little operator training. The examination of 50–60 spermatozoa, which may be an excessive number, required only 15–20 minutes, thus allowing a number of individual samples to be screened in a relatively short time.

Correlation of the computer velocity measurements with those made using timed exposure photography of dark ground images showed good agreement between the two methods (correlation coefficient = 85%; regression coefficient = 1.02). Allowing for sampling variation these results show that the computer technique does not suffer loss of accuracy by its rapidity.

4

Of the 55 semen samples examined during this study, 45 were regarded as 'fertile' on the basis of the zona-free hamster egg penetration assay. These samples gave penetration rates of 10–100%. The remaining ten samples which gave zero or < 10% penetration rates were regarded as an 'infertile' group. There are good grounds to justify these classifications[2] although the technique is not completely reliable.

The mean ($\pm$SE) sperm velocities of the 'fertile' and 'infertile' groups were 36.57 ± 0.26 and 26.78 ± 0.45 $\mu m\,s^{-1}$ respectively. Student's t test showed these means to be significantly different ($p<0.05$). The frequency diagrams representing this data are shown in Figure 1. Statistical analysis using a χ^2 test of normality showed that the sperm velocities within each sample were normally distributed. The within-sample coefficients of variation were consistently in the region of 20%, although five unexplained exceptions (>30%) were found. There was no difference between the two groups in this respect.

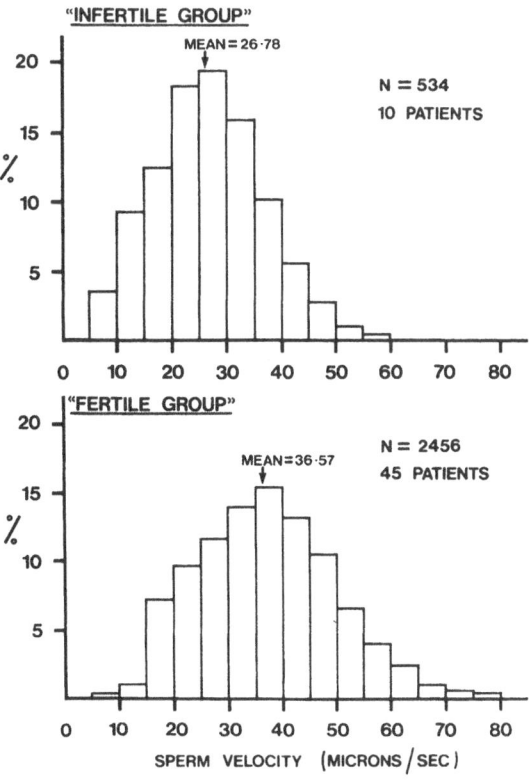

Figure 1 Frequency diagrams of mean sperm velocity in 'infertile' and 'fertile' groups

When the cumulative normal distributions of velocity data for the two groups are plotted on the same axes, the resulting graph is of some interest for its potential predictive value (Figure 2). The intersection between the two curves, which falls in the region of 30 μm s^{-1}, suggests that success in the ovum penetration test may be correlated with sperm velocity. As the sample means increase above 30 μm s^{-1} the probability of correctly identifying a 'fertile' individual rises steeply. The converse is also true.

Examination of the individual sample means of the 55 patients in this study supports this proposal. It was found that 36 out of 45 (77%) samples in the fertile group showed mean velocities greater than 30 μm s^{-1}, whilst 9 out of 10 of the samples in the infertile group showed mean velocities below 30 μm s^{-1}. It is recognized that the examination of further samples is required for the validation of this predictive model; however, an approach such as this may be of considerable value, especially if correlations with other semen parameters are also considered.

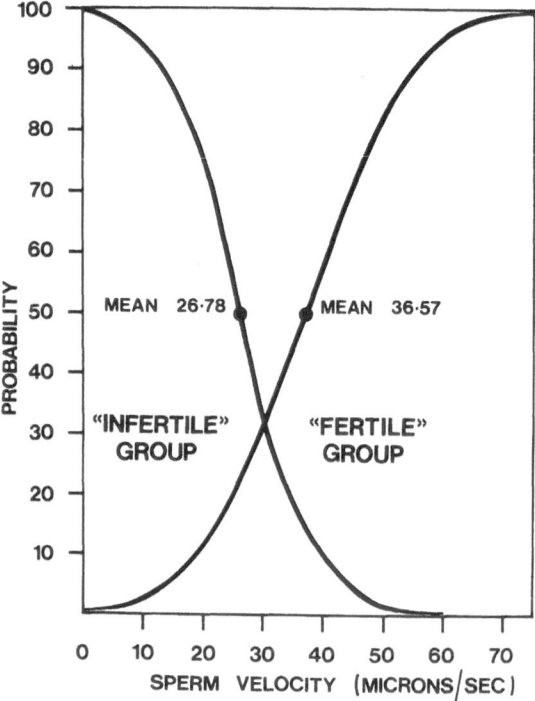

Figure 2 Cumulative normal distributions of mean sperm velocity in 'infertile' and 'fertile' groups

References

1. Emmens, C.W. (1947). The motility and viability of rabbit spermatozoa at different hydrogen-ion concentrations. *J. Physiol.* (Lond.), **106**, 471
2. Overstreet, J.W. (1981). Evaluation of sperm function by tests of sperm ovum interaction *in vitro*. In Spira, A. and Jouannet, P. (eds.) *Human Fertility Factors*, INSERM Symposium Vol. **103**, pp. 263–80 (Paris: INSERM)
3. Moore, H.D.M. (1981). An assessment of the fertilizing ability of spermatozoa in the epididymis of the marmoset monkey (*Callithrix jacchus*). *Int. J. Androl.*, **4**, 321
4. Tyler, J.P.P., Pryor, J.P. and Collins, W.P. (1981). Heterologous ovum penetration by human spermatozoa. *J. Reprod. Fertil.*, **63**, 499

2
Automatic analysis of sperm characteristics by means of a microcomputer system

M. HAZAMA, H. OKADA, O. MATSUMOTO, S. KAMIDONO
and J. ISHIGAMI

INTRODUCTION

Semen analysis is important in evaluating human male fertility, but the subjectivity of the evaluation of sperm characteristics, especially motility, has troubled investigators for many years. Therefore, we have developed a bilevel picture processing system (called the BPP system), using a microcomputer for automatic, objective and quantitative evaluation of sperm characteristics.

MATERIALS AND METHODS

This BPP system consists of a TV camera attached to a phase contrast microscope, two TV monitors, a digitizer tablet, a frame memory, a floppy disk, a printer and a microcomputer that controls them. The interactive software was written mainly in FORTH language and partly in Assembler language (Figure 1).

To begin, well-mixed undiluted semen is inserted into a Makler's 10 μm thick chamber, which is put on the stage of a phase contrast microscope. The picture of sperm appears on the TV monitor (1) with the heads brightly illuminated by the phase contrast apparatus. By optimal thresholding the pixels whose grey levels are lighter than the threshold are displayed as white, and those darker than the threshold as black. As a result, the illuminated sperm head appears as a white spot, and the other seminal part including the sperm tail as a black

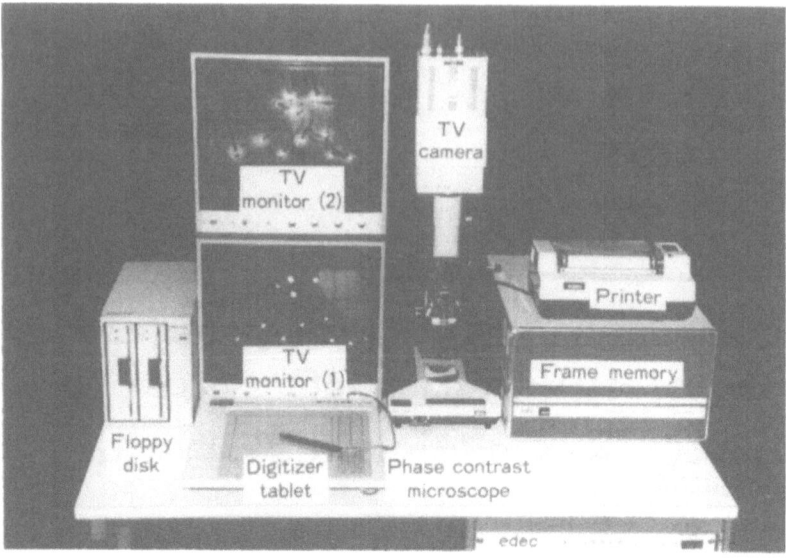

Figure 1 Equipment required for automatic analysis of sperm characteristics by the bi-level picture processing system

background. Ten successive frames taken at intervals of 49.8 ms are stored in the memories to trace the sperm movement for about 0.5 s. The ingredients contained in the semen, such as debris, crystals and other cells cause difficulty here. Some of them appear shining bright like the sperm head. Even if converted to the bi-level picture, they are noted as white spots like the sperm heads and are impossible to distinguish. Therefore, the first frame of the eight-level digital picture in the frame memory which is similar to the original picture, is played back on the TV monitor (2). The data concerning those ingredients are eliminated by inputting their position coordinates through the digitizer tablet with human judgement. In this way X and Y coordinate values of the centroid of each white 'sperm head' on the digital pictures alone are obtained and computed frame by frame. By the criterion of minimum separation the changes of X and Y coordinates of the sperm head give the distance moved between successive frames. By multiplying this distance, the angular velocity of each sperm is computed (Figure 2). However, all sperm that are present in the field of view from the first frame to the final are calculated, but those that swim in or out in latter frames are omitted from the calculation. Determination of the parameters is made on more than 100 sperms in several fields of a single slide, so it is obvious that oligozoospermic specimens require more scans. Within a few minutes the computer supplies a print-out of the results, including the sperm density, the percentage of motile sperm, the mean velocity and the frequency distribution of the velocities. It then stores the data in the floppy disk. Moreover, a dotted outline of each sperm movement is drawn on the TV monitor, by which the pattern of individual sperm movement can be viewed.

RESULTS

Using the BPP system and the new multiple exposure photography method, which we previously reported[1], we estimated sperm characteristics in specimens from 13 infertile males. The data of sperm density, percentage of motile sperm and mean sperm velocity from the two methods were well correlated.

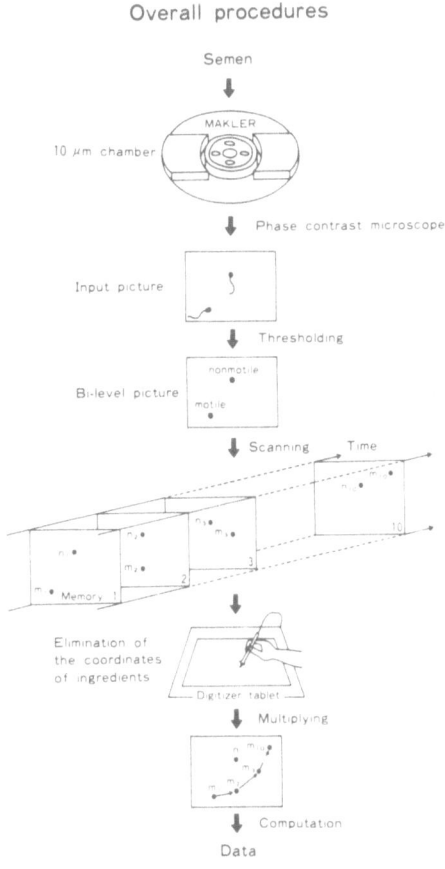

Figure 2 Overall procedures of the bi-level picture processing system

11

DISCUSSION

Various new methodologies assessing sperm motility have been proposed in the last two decades. But an objective, easy to perform and highly informative method has not yet been established. Therefore, we have developed a BPP system as a method comprising both advantages: precision of photographic methods[2] and simplicity of automatic scanning techniques[3].

The merits of this method are objective evaluation of all parameters of semen characteristics with minimum man-hours. It seems the BPP system fulfills most of the requirements of an ideal method of semen analysis. On the other hand, the first of the disadvantages of this method may be that small-sized sperms cannot be detected, as the heads do not shine bright enough under the phase contrast microscope. We are investigating a new picture processing system to detect the sperm tail. Secondly, if two sperms come together, one of them will be excluded from further processing. This occurs only when the sperm density is very high, so suitable dilution of the sperm minimizes this problem[4]. Thirdly, the instrument is rather expensive; however, micro-computers are becoming less expensive, and soon one can be easily afforded.

In conclusion, the BPP system is of great advantage in evaluating sperm characteristics, especially motility, and thus would be a reliable and valuable instrument for clinical diagnosis and research of male infertility.

References

1. Kamidono, S., Hazama, M., Matsumoto, O., Takada, K., Tomioka, O. and Ishigami, J. (1983). Study on human spermatozoal motility: preliminary report on newly developed multiple exposure photography method. *Andrologia*, 15, 111
2. Makler, A. (1978). A new multiple exposure photography method for human spermatozoal motility determination. *Fertil. Steril.*, 30, 192
3. Lee, W.I. and Blandau, R.J. (1979). Laser light scattering study of the effect of progesterone on sperm motility. *Fertil. Steril.*, 32, 320
4. Liu, Y.T. and Warme, P.K. (1977). Computerized evaluation of sperm cell motility. *Comput. Biomed. Res.*, 10, 127

3
In vitro cross penetration testing in infertile couples

U. BRAUN, T. KATZORKE and D. PROPPING

INTRODUCTION

Knowledge of the viability and migration of spermatozoa through cervical mucus is important to the clinician interested in the management of infertility. The evaluation of the sperm–mucus interaction should take place in the pre-ovulatory phase of the menstrual cycle. The *in vitro* Sperm-Penetration-Meter test (SPM-test), first described by Kremer *et al*[1], is a valuable tool for the diagnosis and treatment of infertility, for basic research on sperm transport in the human female, and also useful in order to know whether artificial insemination has a reasonable chance in achieving pregnancy and to know which type of insemination is to be preferred.

MATERIALS AND METHODS

The ability of spermatozoa to penetrate preovulatory cervical mucus (CM) was investigated in 57 infertile couples using the *in vitro* test system (SPM-test). In addition, routine crossover testing was instituted using optimal semen or cervical mucus. The cervical factor of the wives was optimized by ethinyl-oestradiol 0.2 mg/day for 7 days. After 5 days (cycle day 11) the postcoital test was performed, and the cervical mucus collected 2 days later (cycle day 13). For the threefold testing system the samples of mucus were usually used within 24 hours of collection. The male participants were asked to abstain from intercourse for at least 48 hours. The semen was then obtained by masturbation. The ejaculate was analysed within 1 hour of collection to determine sperm

density, % normal morphology, % motility and semen volume. The preparations of the capillary method and the assessment of the SPM-test were carried
out as proposed by Kremer[2].

RESULTS

Figure 1 represents the results of the SPM-test in the threefold testing system,
and their distribution according to the classification described by Kremer[2].
The investigations indicate a normal sperm–mucus interaction in 32 cases
(56%) of the infertile couples and in 43 cases (75%) in the crossover testing
system, when the semen of a fertile donor was used. No difference could be
found in the sperm–mucus interaction between the CM of the wife and that of
a donor, where the husband's semen was employed. No penetration at all
occurred in 13 cases, which was due to a female factor in eight tests, as the
crossover testing shows. No good correlation could be found between the PCT
and the SPM-test. From a total of 43 tests, 63% have shown corresponding
results in both testing systems when the poor postcoital tests were included,
and only 51% when these tests were omitted.

As the sperm–mucus interaction depends on the semen quality as well as the
cervical mucus, investigations were performed on both the partners, and the
SPM-test was examined. For the male, the results have shown that the test
becomes worse as the semen quality decreases.

The working female diagnosis (Figure 2) showed: no pathology in 29 cases,

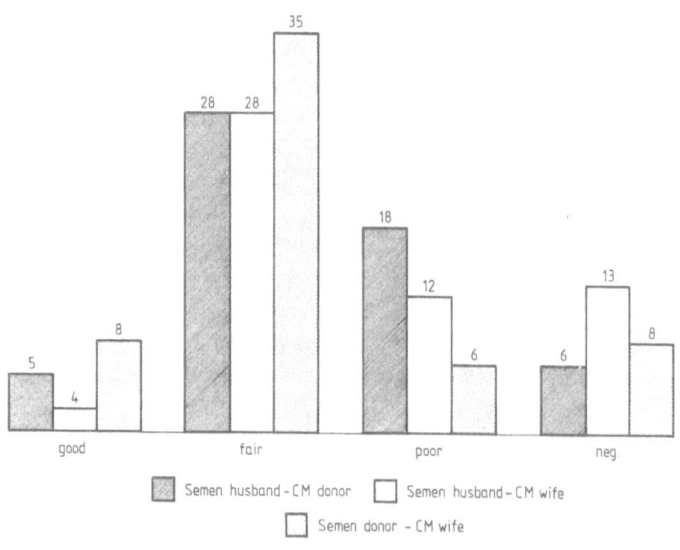

Figure 1

14

an anatomical factor in 7 cases, an hormonal factor in 15 cases, an hormonal and a cervical factor in two cases, a cervical factor in one case and endo-metriosis in one. From a total of 29 cases with no pathology nearly 50% have shown a disturbed sperm–mucus interaction in which six cases were due to a cervical factor and 7 due to a male factor, as could be seen in the crossover testing system. 50% of the cases, where an hormonal factor was assumed to be the cause of infertility, have shown a disturbed sperm–mucus interaction. As the crossover testing system shows, only a third can be attributed to the hormonal factor. In the other cases a male factor may be responsible for the bad result. The anatomical factor seems to have no influence on the sperm–mucus interaction.

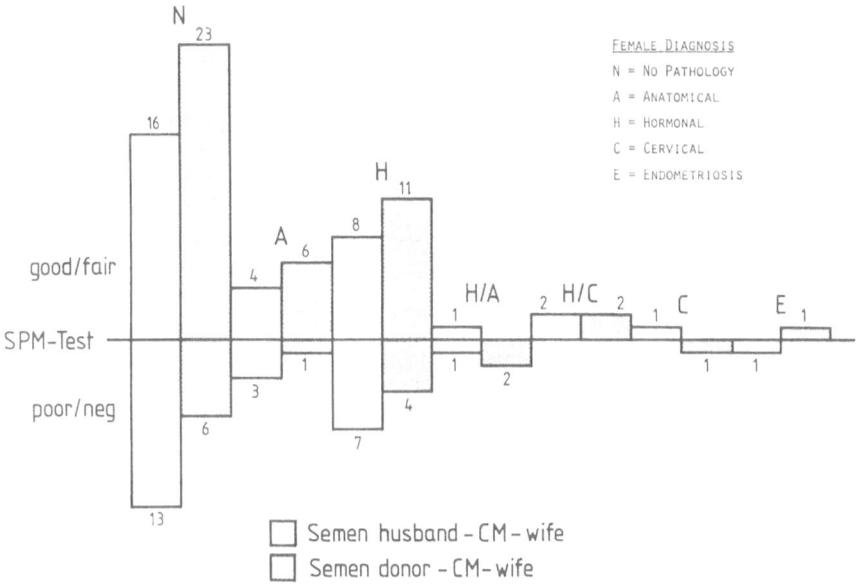

Figure 2

Figure 3 shows the main contributing infertility factor in the couples before and after the SPM-test. The investigations indicate, that the working diagnosis is in only a few cases responsible for the disturbed sperm–mucus interaction, and that a shifting in the diagnosis has taken place. 'Unexplained' means that the SPM-test has given a good/fair result, and that further investigations are necessary to evaluate the reason for infertility.

The results of the threefold testing system are summarized in Table 1. The preferred treatment is described according to the results of the SPM-test.

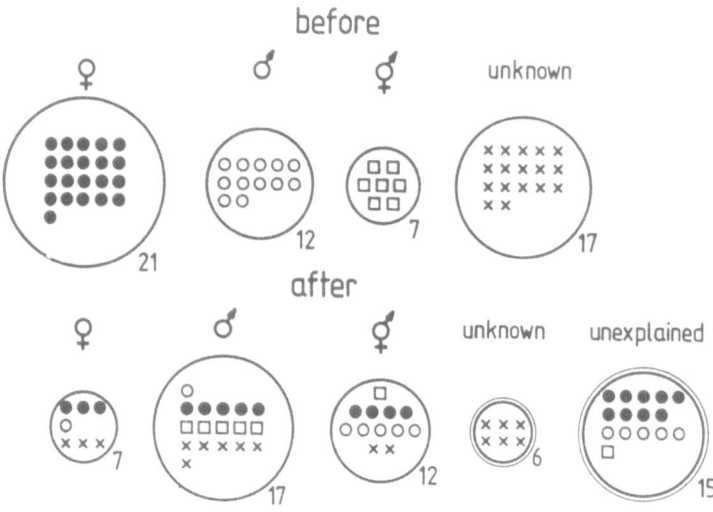

Figure 3

Table 1 Results of the cross SPM-test and possible treatment of infertility

	Results of SPM-test			Treatment
	♀●♂	♀○♂	♀●♂	
1.	+	+	+	Optimizing of cervical mucus
2.	+	–	+	AID; IU AIH (?)
3.	–	–	+	AID; HOP-test; IU AIH (?)
4.	+	–	–	IU AIH
5.	–	–	–	[IU AIH] ?; Embryotransfer?

♀●♂ = CM-donor; semen husband

♀○♂ = CM-wife; semen husband

♀●♂ = CM-wife; semen donor

References

1. Kremer, J. (1965). A simple sperm penetration test. *Int. J. Fertil.*, **10**, 201
2. Kremer, J. (1980). *In vitro* sperm penetration in cervical mucus and AIH. In Emperaire, J. C., Audebert, A. and Hafez, E. S. E. (eds.) *Homologous Artificial Insemination (AIH) Clinics in Andrology*. Vol. I, p. 30. (The Hague/Boston/London: Martinus Nijhoff)

4
A new standardized *in vitro* penetration test (bovine) measuring the capacity of fertilization. I

GY. CORRADI, G. GIMES, I. SÜLE and F. BALOGH

INTRODUCTION

In the general examination of the infertile man it is no longer sufficient to diagnose the capacity of fertilization of sperm from data obtained by observing the classical parameters (concentration, motility%, etc.). The andrologists have long been seeking a new general method which would show the functional value of the sperm, in contradiction to those static parameters which have previously been used. For this reason the post-coital test[1], the *in vitro* capillary test[2], and the standardized human penetration test[3] are now suggested for diagnostic purposes. It is obvious that the previous two tests have real diagnostic value, but their technique needs a well organized and often rather a difficult preparation. To observe sperm penetration in human mucus is often not easy because in the anovulatory cycle and in cases of cervicitis mucus of proper quality is not present. The penetration tests with human mucus needs the close cooperation of the andrologist and gynaecologist in order to obtain evaluable results. Therefore we have devised a standardized *in vitro* sperm penetration test, where the penetration agent was the cervical mucus of the cow (BCM).

MATERIALS AND METHODS

The bovine cervical mucus was collected by a skilled veterinary at the Central Hungarian Animal Insemination Station. The cow produces a great quantity

17

of mucus prior to ovulation which runs down the legs of the animal; the ovaries are palpable at the time of ovulation during rectal examination. To select the proper animals needs great care, because the not clear and transparent mucus indicates cervicitis and has an unfavourable effect on the penetration test. The mucus, from six cows, was aspirated into plastic capillary tubes, 120 mm long and 1 mm internal diameter, and the tubes stored in liquid nitrogen.

Samples of semen were obtained by masturbation from healthy male donors attending the andrological out-patient department, who had abstained from sexual activity for at least 5 days. After collection the semen was divided in two. In one aliquot we measured the quantity and traditional andrological parameters. The other aliquot of semen was used for the bovine penetration test. We performed two parallel examinations in every case. The various parameters of the sperm we used are shown in Table 1.

The parameters used in the diagnosis of the mucus, i.e. spinnbarkeit and ferning, showed +3 in every case. We compared the physical characteristics of the mucus stored in liquid nitrogen for 3, 6, 9 and 12 months, but we observed no reduction in quality. The mucus from one animal filled 100 plastic tubes to a height of 70–80 mm. Overflow of the mucus was prevented by thick cotton at the tip and by soldering the other end.

RESULTS

We started our examinations with the slide drop method, where a drop of bovine cervical mucus was mixed with a drop of semen. Sperm motility could be observed in bovine cervical mucus after 5 hours under the microscope. Their marked orientation and unidirectional motion was outstanding during the first 60 minutes. During penetration, phalanx formation could be observed[4]. The characteristic of sperm motility in bovine mucus is identical with that in human mucus, which excludes immunological immobilization[5,6]. After these results we performed capillary tube penetration tests at room temperature. The plastic tubes were placed into small test tubes which contained 1 ml semen. We changed the angular offset of the system between

Table 1 Sperm quality of the semen used in the penetration test

	Mean	$\pm SD$
Concentration /ml	43×10^6	5.1
Motility %	80.2	3.15
Intensive motility %	56.0	7.02
Morphologically normal %	74.4	9.08
Fructose mmol/l	17.1	2.98

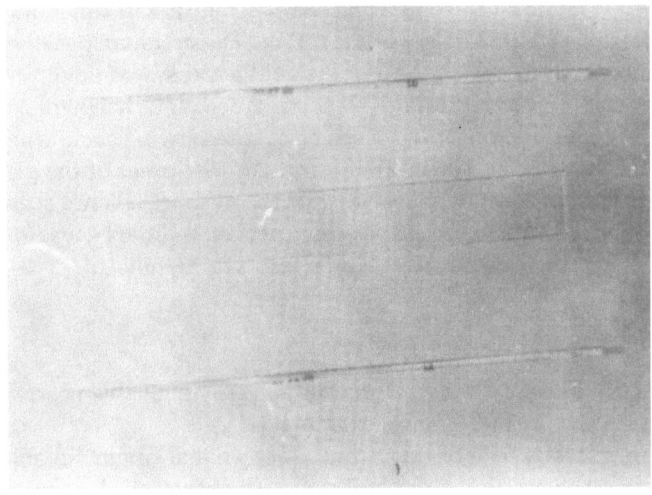

Figure 1   Tubes under the light microscope

5–90 degrees and the period of penetration from 10 to 180 minutes. Readings were performed by light microscope with ×100 magnification. The plastic tube is transparent so it can be examined with no difficulty (Figure 1). The measure of distance of penetration was given by a glass-plate which had a scale on it (Figure 2). In accordance with our serial experiments the best angular

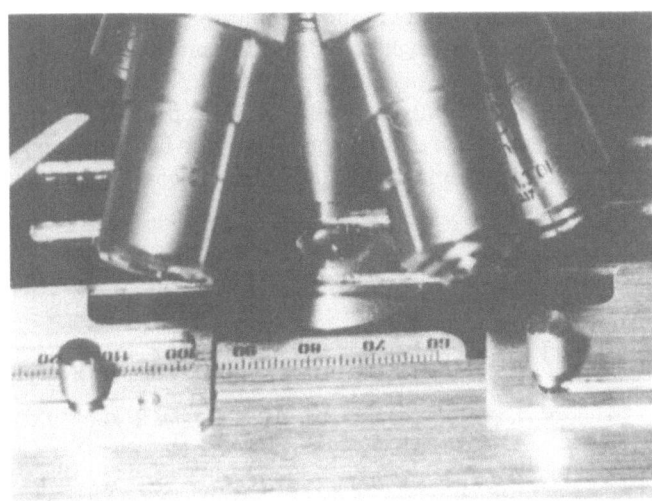

Figure 2   Plastic capillary tubes containing bovine cervical mucus and the glass plate with scale

offset was 30° to the horizontal line, as the mucus did not flow up thus ensuring the upwards movement of the sperm. The optimum penetration time was 60 minutes during which the motility of the sperm was unidirectional. In the case of normal sperm we found 1-2 spermatozoas at a height of 70-80 mm. When the test time was longer we observed sperms moving back, which meant that their motion was no longer unidirectional. The result of the penetration test is given as a value which shows the furthest distance where a spermatozoa could be found. In 140 cases the average penetration distance was 75 ± 5 mm. The correlation between the two parallel tests was significant.

DISCUSSION

The aim of our research was to work out an easily available penetration test which is necessary in andrological examinations.

It seemed obvious to look for a mucus of animal origin suitable for the penetration test. Several authors found that the penetration value of human sperm in bovine mucus is almost the same as the values obtained from human mucus[4,5,7]. The motility of the spermatozoa in bovine cervical mucus was unidirectional upwards in the first 60 minutes.

The molecular structure of human and bovine mucus was investigated using laser light scattering spectroscopy, and it showed that the structure of the macromolecules of both samples are similar[8].

Our examinations show that mucus can be stored for as long as a year in liquid nitrogen and that it preserves its structure and function after thawing[7,9].

On the basis of our results we found that mucus should be aspirated into the plastic capillary tube to a height of 70-80 mm, and that the penetration test should be performed at 30° angular offset. At 30° the sperm penetrates as in a counter-current, and in this way we may approach the physiological conditions. Results of our research show that our bovine penetration test is suitable for practical examinations, and may become a useful method in andrological practice.

References

1. Baruch, A.L., Yedwab, G., David, P.M., Hommonai, Z.T. and Paz, G.F. (1983). Establishment of a method for preservation of human cervical mucus *in vitro* penetration test. *Gynecol. Obstet. Invest.*, **15**, 254
2. Kremer, J. (1965). A simple method of penetration test. *Int. J. Fertil.*, **10**, 201
3. Gimes, R. (1982). A funkcionalis meddöség diagnózisa és therapiája a spermapenetració tökrében. *PhD Thesis*, Hungary.
4. Gaddum-Rosse, P., Blandau, P.J. and Lee, W.I. (1980). Sperm penetration into cervical mucus *in vitro* I. Comparative studies. *Fertil. Steril.*, **33**, 636
5. Gaddum-Rosse, P., Blandau, P.J. and Lee, W.I. (1980). Sperm penetration into cervical mucus *in vitro* II. Human spermatozoa in bovine mucus. *Fertil. Steril.*, **33**, 644

6. Moghissi, S. K., Segal, S. and Meinhold, D. B. C. (1982). *In vitro* sperm penetration: studies in human and bovine cervical mucus. *Fertil. Steril.*, **37**, 823
7. Bergman, A., Amit, A., David, M. A., Hommonai, Z. T. and Paz, G. (1981). Penetration of human ejaculated spermatozoa into human and bovine cervical mucus I. Correlation between penetration values. *Fertil. Steril.*, **36**, 363
8. Lee, W. I., Verdugo, P., Blandau, R. J. and Gaddum Rosse, P. (1977). Molecular arrangement of cervical mucus: a re-evaluation based on laser light scattering spectroscopy. *Gynecol. Invest.*, **8**, 254
9. Broer, K. H. (1981). Diagnostik und Therapie zervikaler Sterilitätsursachen. In Kaiser, R. (ed.) *Menschlicher Fortpflanzung.* pp. 202–19 (Stuttgart, New York: Thieme Verlag)
10. Corradi, Gy., Gimes, G., Süle, I. and Balogh, F. (1983). A new standardized *in vitro* penetration test (bovine) measuring the capacity of fertilization I. In this volume.

5
A new standardized *in vitro* penetration test (bovine) measuring the capacity of fertilization. II

G. GIMES, GY. CORRADI and F. BALOGH

INTRODUCTION

We have described the technical details of the standardized *in vitro* penetration test with bovine mucus in a previous study[10]. In this study we have examined the penetration ability of sperm in bovine cervical mucus aspirated in capillary tubes and stored in liquid nitrogen.

MATERIAL AND METHODS

To establish the normal penetration distance we used ejaculate from 20 normal donors. Traditional andrological examinations were performed on one aliquot of the semen. The other aliquot was used for bovine penetration tests. We then investigated the semen of 50 andrologically abnormal patients. Statistical examinations of our results were made with the help of R-20 type computer with the BMDP statistical program. We applied two kinds of statistical measuring: correlation between the traditional and new variables, and Cluster analysis on the basis of the variables and the individual cases.

RESULTS

In 12 cases of 50 abnormal patients the penetration test was normal or near normal – although they would have been characterized abnormal by traditional andrologic methods. This group was separated and termed 'special group'.

The analysis made on the basis of the correlation of the seven variables (concentration per ml, motility %, intensive motility %, morphologically normal %, initial fructose mmol/l, penetrational distance I and II), produced the following results (Table 1).

Table 1   Correlation between penetration values and traditional parameters

Parameter	Normal group	Abnormal group	Special group
Concentration	0.221	0.557	0.630
Motility (%)	0.040	0.578	0.298
Intensive motility (%)	0.027	0.569	0.219
Morphologically normal (%)	0.181	0.401	0.159
Fructose mmol/l	0.152	0.129	0.444

Motility and intensive motility – significant correlation.
Penetration distance I and II   – significant correlation.
Concentration, motility and
    intensive motility   – good correlation.

The correlation counting revealed that the penetration distance correlates well with traditional variables, except for the initial fructose levels. The mean values shown that the average penetration distance is 76 mm in the normal group and that the deviation is small (Table 2). In the abnormal group the mean is 54 mm SD±21 mm. In the special group the distance is 70 mm SD±8 mm.

DISCUSSION

The lower limit of the new variable (penetration distance) is given by the special patients group, below which, in all probability, the patients are

Table 2   Mean±SD of the parameters

Parameter	Normal group	Abnormal group	Special group
Penetration value	7.6±0.5	5.4±2.1	7.0±0.8
Concentration	44.0±5.5	22.1±11.0	21.8±6.5
Motility	83.2±3.3	66.9±13.6	74.6±8.8
Intensive motility	59.0±7.1	33.8±14.4	45.2±11.9
Morphologically normal	76.8±9.3	51.4±18.9	57.3±11.6

abnormal, above it they are normal. If the traditional variable is lower, then the new variable correlates better than the traditional ones. Cluster analysis revealed that our new variable (penetration distance) correlates well to the concentration, motility and the intensive motility. It does not correlate well to the rate of normal cells and to the initial fructose values, which do not correlate well with each other. In summary, we can often say that the normal and abnormal cases can be separated from each other with great assurances by the sperm penetration test.

The so-called special group is interesting from the point of view of the normal values. Those patients belong to this category where a weaker capacity of fertilization was registered by parameters of the traditional andrological methods, and normal or near normal values were obtained by the penetration test. We followed up case records of these patients, and we learned that pregnancy occurred in 6 out of 12 cases. We have no information in two cases, and in four cases we found problems in the wife. The number of pregnancies is high, and are much higher than in the group of abnormal patients.

These results stimulate us to examine the special group of patients in greater numbers, because the *in vitro* penetration test appears to be more informative than other *in vitro* tests, and more properly reflects the expected chance of fertilization.

The examination of patients with a low fertilization potential shows a significant correlation between the decrease in penetrational distance and the weakened capacity of fertilization. The penetrational distance appears to be a favourable sign of fertility.

These examinations allow us to conclude that the *in vitro* penetration test, performed with standardized bovine mucus in a plastic capillary tube, is an appropriate complementory method of measuring fertility.

The main advantages of our bovine penetration test as compared to other methods are:

(1) The necessary quantity of bovine mucus can be obtained without limits.
(2) It can be stored in liquid nitrogen for a long time.
(3) It can be used at any time, and the cervical mucus is standardized.

The results of our penetration tests depend exclusively on the quality of the ejaculate.

References

1. Baruch, A. L., Yedwab, G., David, P. M., Hommonai, Z. T. and Paz, G. F. (1983). Establishment of a method for preservation of human cervical mucus *in vitro* penetration test. *Gynecol. Obstet. Invest.*, 15, 254
2. Kremer, J. (1965). A simple method of penetration test. *Int. J. Fertil.*, 10, 201

3. Gimes, R. (1982). A funkcionalis meddöség diagnózisa és therapiája a spermapenetració tökrében. *PhD Thesis*, Hungary.
4. Gaddum-Rosse, P., Blandau, P. J. and Lee, W. I. (1980). Sperm penetration into cervical mucus *in vitro* I. Comparative studies. *Fertil. Steril.*, **33**, 636
5. Gaddum-Rosse, P., Blandau, P. J. and Lee, W. I. (1980). Sperm penetration into cervical mucus *in vitro* II. Human spermatozoa in bovine mucus. *Fertil. Steril.*, **33**, 644
6. Moghissi, S. K., Segal, S. and Meinhold, D. B. C. (1982). *In vitro* sperm penetration: studies in human and bovine cervical mucus. *Fertil. Steril.*, **37**, 823
7. Bergman, A., Amit, A., David, M. A., Hommonai, Z. T. and Paz, G. (1981). Penetration of human ejaculated spermatozoa into human and bovine cervical mucus I. Correlation between penetration values. *Fertil. Steril.*, **36**, 363
8. Lee, W. I., Verdugo, P., Blandau, R. J. and Gaddum Rosse, P. (1977). Molecular arrangement of cervical mucus: a re-evaluation based on laser light scattering spectroscopy. *Gynecol. Invest.*, **8**, 254
9. Broer, K. H. (1981). Diagnostik und Therapie zervikaler Sterilitätsursachen. In Kaiser, R. (ed.) *Menschlicher Fortpflanzung.* pp. 202–19 (Stuttgart, New York: Thieme Verlag)
10. Corradi, Gy., Gimes, G., Süle, I. and Balogh, F. (1983). A new standardized *in vitro* penetration test (bovine) measuring the capacity of fertilization I. In this volume.

6
Penetration of zona-free hamster eggs by human spermatozoa. Comparison of two methods

M. GELAS, E. WAREMBOURG, B. SELE, C. OSTO RERO,
C. ESTRADE and P. JALBERT

INTRODUCTION

Standard semen analysis is an imprecise method of determining male infertility. The human spermatozoa – hamster ova *in vitro* fertilization system, first described by Yanagimachi[1], has been proposed for this aim. In the present study the use of an *in vitro* fertilization assay employing zona-free hamster eggs has several aims.

The first is to obtain a direct chromosomal analysis of the human spermatozoa, as initially reported by Rudak[2]. The interest in obtaining this has been emphasized by Boue *et al*[3]. They show that 50% of human fertilized eggs, resulting from a spermatozoan penetration, have an abnormal chromosomal pattern.

The addition of a human *in vitro* fertilization (IVF) programme could be useful as a selective test for IVF donors or as a diagnostic test for unexplained sterility. The same test could possibly be used as a means of testing the sperms resistance to *in vitro* processing.

Eighty zona-free hamster egg assays were performed from July, 1982 to June, 1983. Fifteen thousand oocytes were treated, and 100 sperms tested during this period.

The testing of two mediums, concurrently, for a great number of these assays forms the original part of this study, the 'hamsters' test being largely used by other teams of workers[4,5]. The first medium or the

Biggers–Whitten–Whittingham medium (BWW) is a classic one for this test[6]. The second one is the French Menezo medium or B_2 used in human IVF cultures.

MATERIALS AND METHODS

Semen donors

Semen donors form two groups. The first group is formed by experimental donors or volunteers. The second one is formed by men whose wives belong to the human IVF programme. In this second group infertility is due to tubal obstruction in the wife, associated or not with mixed hypofertility or unexplained sterility. In the two groups some of the men proved their fertility by having fathered a child.

Sperm processing

After a period of sexual abstinence, of at least 48 hours, semen samples are collected from donors at the laboratory and allowed to liquify for 30 minutes at room temperature.

An aliquot of the semen sample is taken for traditional semen analysis. In the first method using BWW medium, 1 ml of the remaining sperm is diluted with 10 ml of the solution and filtered through sterile paper tissues. The sample is centrifuged at 600 g for 10 minutes. The sperm pellet is washed and centrifuged twice more at 600 g for 5 minutes, and then resuspended in BWW medium to give a final concentration of 10^7 sperm/ml. The motility is again evaluated. Droplets (100 μl) of this sperm solution are placed under paraffin oil in sterile petri dishes – the dishes are incubated at 37 °C in 5% CO_2 for 5–7 hours to allow for capacitation.

The second method using Menezo B_2 medium differs, first by the sperm dilution: 0.275 ml of the liquified sperm is diluted with only 2.5 ml of B_2. The sample is then centrifuged at 200 g for 10 minutes twice only. The final pellet is resuspended in B_2 to give an equal concentration of 10^7 sperm/ml and the motility evaluated.

The main difference between the two methods appears at this stage, the B_2 sperm is kept for 5 hours in ambient air at room temperature – the B_2 droplets are made after 5 hours just before receiving the eggs.

Egg processing

Eggs are obtained from female golden hamsters. The hyperstimulation consists of an intraperitoneal injection of 50 IU of pregnant mare serum at 10 a.m. on the day of their post-oestral discharge. 50 IU of human Chorionic Gonado-tropin are given on day 3 at 11 p.m. Animals are killed at 4 p.m. Dissection of their oviduct releases the cumulus; the cumulus is dissociated by hyaluronidase. Eggs are washed and then put in trypsin for 1 min to remove the zona pellucida and washed again. Four hamsters are used for each experiment. Ten to fifteen zona-free eggs are placed in each sperm droplet in BWW medium or Menezo medium. They are incubated at 37 °C with 5% CO_2 and 95% humidity for 2–14 hours.

Fertilization check

After 2–5 hours, 25 eggs per medium or 50 eggs per sperm are examined with a phase-contrast microscope.

RESULTS

Interpretation of the check test

The first point to emphasize is that with the 'hamster' test there may be difficulties of interpretation. Non-fertilized eggs with only the first polar body or the germinal vesicle can be easily eliminated. Special attention must be paid to borderline pictures. Eggs with more than two pronuclei can be considered as activated. But eggs with a single pronucleus and a polar body, or eggs with the spindle of the polar body raise problems.

It is not impossible that these pictures correspond to fertilization stages and are important in explaining sperm failure. For instance, three sorts of pictures are considered as fertilized eggs:

(1) A swollen sperm head with or without a polar body,
(2) Two pronuclei with or without the tail of the fertilizing spermatozoa, and
(3) Pictures of polyspermia with several swollen sperm heads.

Fertilization rates/fertility

The study of the fertilization rate in the two groups: proven fertility and unproven fertility of this population (Table 1) shows that the test is even more effective for unproven fertility – there is of course a statistical bias, the IVF group probably contains a lot of very fertile men.

Fertilization rates/sperm motility and numeration

The quality of the sperm can be used to separate sperms: a sperm being con-

29

Table 1 Fertilization rate/fertility

	Fertilized eggs	Unfertilized eggs	Total
Proven fertility	68 (10.9%)	556	624
Unproven fertility	198 (17.0%)	964	1162

χ^2-test, $p = 0.005$

Table 2 Fertilization rate/sperm motility

	Fertilization rate	
	< 20%	> 20%
Deficient sperms	8	1
Good sperms	40	15

not significant by modified χ^2-test
Deficient sperms: motility < 50% forward progression N < 20×10^6/ml

sidered as deficient if the numeration is inferior to 20×10^6/ml and the motility inferior to 50% (Table 2). No significant difference can be found between good sperm and deficient sperm for the fertilization rate. This test does not give a very good rate of reproductibility, even for good sperms.

Comparison of the two sperm processing methods

The Biggers medium (BWW) is a very simple one, with the addition of human serum albumin; but the final solution has to be prepared from the stock solution just before the assay – the Menezo medium (B_2) is a very rich one, but is ready to use from the commercial solution, containing bovine serum albumin and essential amino-acids.

Survival test in the two methods

The survival study tests the difference between the initial motility of the sperm

Table 3 Survival test BWW versus B_2 medium

	Test $\oplus$
BWW	20/45 (44.4%)
B_2	18/45 (40.0%)

differences are not significant in paired series
Survival test $\oplus$ motility decrease after sperm preparation < 20%

and the motility just before insemination. The survival test is positive if this difference is inferior to 20% (Table 3).

The impression is that B_2 medium favours deficient sperms – however, no significant difference is found between the two methods.

Fertilization rates in the two methods

The study of the fertilization rate also shows no significant difference between the two methods (Table 4). B_2 Menezo medium does not improve the fertilization rate, but is equally good for a fertilization check.

Table 4 Fertilization rate in BWW versus B_2 medium

	Fertilized eggs	Unfertilized eggs
BWW	93	636
B_2	92	572

not significant by χ^2-test

Variation of the contact-time for one sperm

An experimental donor with a very good proven fertility was tested several times. The pre-incubation time and especially the contact-time between the two gametes varied from 2 to 5 hours.

This sperm numeration and motility each time falls in a very close range (70–85% motility, 80–100×10^6 = numeration).

Figure 1 shows two contrasting results; the first curve, with very poor fertilization rates, is probably due to non-respect of the collection conditions, e.g. sexual abstinence. The second curve shows an increase in the fertilization rate with the contact-time.

From one day to another, this good sperm can take longer or less time to penetrate the ova. Bad results with good sperms could be explained by too short a contact-time or too short a pre-incubation time. This point must be verified by other experiments.

DISCUSSION

For the two methods used in our assays no significant difference was found in sperm motility, survival and fertilization rate. The Menezo B_2 method is, nevertheless, a very simple one and represents a good test for human IVF.

This heterospecific 'hamster' test shows a wide range of fertilization rates

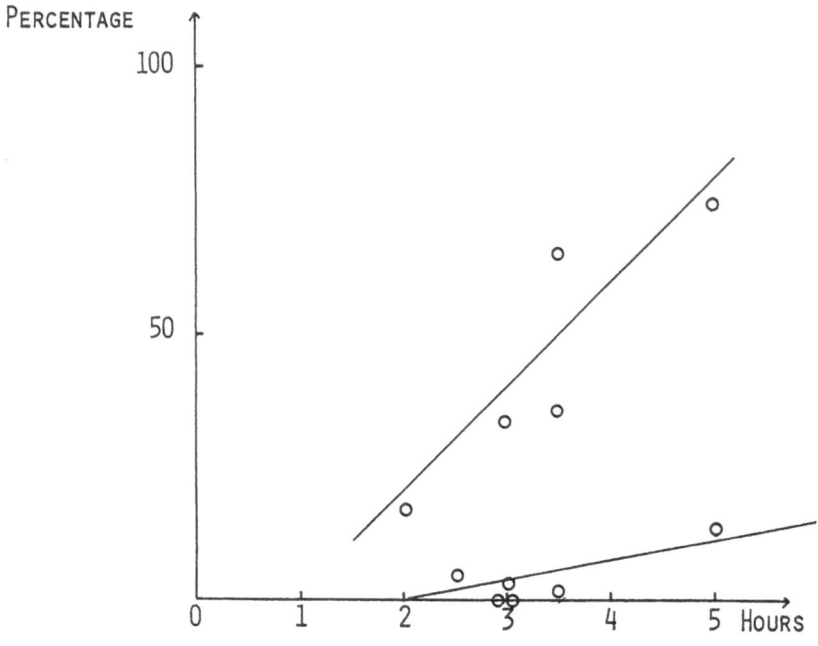

Figure 1   Variation in contact-time on the percentage fertilization rate

even for good sperms (fertilization rate 18.3% ±SD 23.5). There is no obvious correlation between motility, clinical fertility and fertilization rates, the interpretation of the test is still disturbed by borderline pictures. In the full meaning of a diagnostic test this is not a reproducible method.

In conclusion, this test cannot be used as a selecting test for IVF or artificial insemination donors, but it shows a good degree of repetition for sperm resistance before a human IVF.

However, this test must be carried out to detect a male factor in an infertile group, especially with normal semen characteristics. In any case it remains the first step in obtaining the human spermatozoan karyotype.

References

1. Yanagimachi, R., Yanagimachi, H. and Rogers, B.J. (1976). *J. Biol. Reprod.*, **15**, 471–6
2. Rudak, E., Jacobs, P.A. and Yanagimachi, R. (1978). *Nature*, **274**, 911–13
3. Boue, J., Boue, H. and Lazar, P. (1975). *Teratology*, **12**, 11–26
4. Rogers, B.J., Van Campen, H., Ueno, M., Lambert, H., Bronson, R. and Hale, R. (1979). *Fertil. Steril.*, **32**, 664–70
5. Banos, C., Gonzales, G., Herrera, E., Buston-Obregon, E. (1979). *Anchologia*, **11**, 197
6. Biggers, J.D., Whitten, W.R. and Whittingham, ? (1971). In Daniel, J.C. (ed.) *Methods in Mammalian Embryology.* p. 86. (San Francisco: Freeman)

7
Reduced penetration of zona-free hamster ova by cryopreserved human spermatozoa

D. NAVOT, E. J. MARGALIOTH, N. LAUFER
and J. G. SCHENKER

The use of frozen semen for AID has gained wide acceptance, because of the relatively simple cryopreserving technique and the increased flexibility this method offers any donor insemination programme. Storage of frozen semen is even more important for the preservation of future fertility of young men who face permanent injury to spermatogenesis due to irradiation or chemotherapy for malignant diseases. Pregnancy occurs in 60–90% of women inseminated with freshly ejaculated semen from a donor[1]. Unfortunately, the conception rate with frozen semen remains about 50–60%[2]. This reduced pregnancy rate has been associated with morphological and biochemical changes as well as a 30–50% drop in motile spermatozoa of frozen–thawed semen[3]. With the introduction of the 'human sperm penetration into zona free hamster ova' test the assessment of the fertilizing potential of human spermatozoa has been enhanced. The test has been shown to be of superior predictive value when compared with the standard semen analyses[4].

The purpose of the present study was to compare fresh and cryopreserved human semen in regard to their ability to penetrate into zona-free hamster eggs, bearing in mind the reduced fertilization rate with freeze–thawed sperm in clinical practice.

MATERIALS AND METHODS

Ova were harvested from superovulated mature female hamsters. Egg preparation and stripping of the zona were performed by methods described before[5]. Human ejaculates were obtained from 12 medical students between the ages of 29 and 34 years, all of recent proven fertility. Each sample was divided into two equal aliquots: one aliquot to be frozen and the other to be used as a fresh sample.

To the liquified aliquots of 1–1.5 ml semen 10% glycerol (v/v) was added slowly and by continuous stirring. The samples were stored in a liquid nitrogen tank for periods of 3–8 weeks. Samples were then thawed at 37 °C for 20–30 minutes and the sperm prepared for testing according to the procedures described previously[4,5]. All experiments were performed in duplicate for each semen sample. 20–50 eggs were transferred into each sperm drop containing 1×10^6 sperm cells and incubated in 5% CO_2 in air at 37 °C for 6 hours. All ova were fixed overnight with a mixture of methanol and acetic acid (3:1), stained with 1% acetolacmoid and examined under a phase-contrast microscope. The presence of a swollen sperm head or male pronucleus with a visible tail in the cytoplasm was considered positive penetration. 1200 ova were examined by this method. Penetration rate was defined as the number of ova with positive penetration/total number of ova examined $\times 100$, and sperm incorporation as total number of penetrated sperm cells/number of ova with positive penetration. For statistical evaluation of the differences in the parameters examined Student's t test was applied.

RESULTS

Mean sperm volume of the 12 donors' fresh ejaculates was 3.1 ± 0.7 (range 2–7.2 ml). Mean fresh sperm concentration was $102 \pm 51 \times 10^6$ sperm cells ml^{-1} (range 45–$220 \times 10^6\,ml^{-1}$) and mean sperm motility $66 \pm 14\%$ (range 40–85%). Fresh sperm penetrated a mean of $77.8 \pm 19\%$ of the ova (range 56–100%), and the mean sperm cells incorporated per egg was 4.3 ± 3.9 (range 1.3–14.5). Table 1 summarizes the changes in motility penetration rate and sperm incorporation per egg of the individual fresh and cryopreserved semen samples. Motility was decreased in all frozen–thawed samples by 25–89%. Out of the 12 samples 10 showed a decrease in penetration rate of 18–90% while only two samples (No. 3 and 8) maintained the same rate as before cryopreservation.

Sperm incorporation into penetrated ova was reduced in all frozen–thawed samples except one (No. 7). Motility was reduced by $61 \pm 21\%$ ($p < 0.001$), penetration rate by $53 \pm 34\%$ ($p < 0.01$) and sperm incorporation into penetrated ova dropped by $50 \pm 28\%$ ($p < 0.05$).

DISCUSSION

Our study confirms previous observations that a decrease in spermatozoal

Table 1 The effect of cryopreservation on sperm motility, and penetration into zona-free hamster ova of individual samples

Donor	% Motility			% Ova penetration			Sperm/penetration oocyte		
	F	F-T	% decrease	F	F-T	% decrease	F	F-T	% decrease
1	80	40	50	90	23	72	2.6	1.25	51
2	60	21	65	59	31	47	1.8	1.2	33
3	77	25	68	56	57	0	1.6	1.2	25
4	60	14	77	78	0	100	3.7	0	100
5	70	10	86	100	63	37	4.1	1.8	69
6	81	43	47	71	19	73	3.8	2.0	47
7	85	10	88	57	17	70	1.6	1.6	0
8	60	40	33	100	100	0	14.5	7.8	46
9	40	30	25	100	56	44	9.7	1.4	78
10	75	8	89	100	10	90	5.3	1	81
11	50	15	70	61	50	18	2.0	1	50
12	55	30	45	62	8	87	1.3	1	23

F=Fresh; F-T=frozen–thawed.

35

motility is the most striking effect of semen freezing. We found a decrease of 60% in sperm motility which is in accordance with a 50% change shown in other studies[6].

As a whole group the samples examined showed the same general trend of decrease in both motility and ova penetration, but no correlation was found between the rates of decline for these two parameters. This reflects the observation that for an individual sample the post-thaw drop in motility is not followed by a concomitant decrease in penetration rate of a similar degree. In spite of the fact that penetration rate decreased substantially for the group as a whole, 75% of the specimens still maintained a penetration rate exceeding 14% which is thought to be the lower penetration level for fertile semen[4].

It may be concluded from this study that all three parameters examined – sperm motility, penetration rate, and frequency of sperm incorporation – were reduced markedly following cryopreservation. These findings may explain the relative decrease in pregnancy rates following cryopreservation of human sperm.

References

1. Aiman, J. (1982). Factors affecting the success of donor insemination. *Fertil. Steril.*, **37**, 97
2. Steinberger, E. and Smith, K.D. (1973). Artificial insemination with fresh or frozen semen: A comparative study. *J. Am. Med. Assoc.*, **223**, 778
3. Serres, C., Jouannet, P., Czyglick, F. and David, G. (1980). Effects of freezing on spermatozoa motility. In David, G. and Price, W.S. (eds.) *Human Artificial Insemination and Semen Preservation*, p. 147. (New York: Plenum Press)
4. Rogers, B.J., Van Campen, H., Veno, M., Lambert, H., Bronson, K. and Hale, R. (1979). Analysis of human spermatozoal fertilizing ability using zona-free ova. *Fertil. Steril.*, **32**, 64
5. Margalioth, E.J., Laufer, N., Navot, D., Voss, R. and Schenker, J.G. (1983). Reduced fertilization ability of zona-free hamster ova by spermatozoa from male partners of normal infertile couples. *Arch. Androl.*, **10**, 67
6. Smith, K.D. and Steinberger, E. (1973). Survival of spermatozoa in a human sperm bank. *J. Am. Med. Assoc.*, **7**, 774

8
Effect of caffeine on human sperm penetration into zona-free hamster ova

E. J. MARGALIOTH, D. NAVOT, J. Y. MAY, N. LAUFER,
J. OVADIA and J. G. SCHENKER

INTRODUCTION

The exogenous addition of caffeine to human semen has been noted to increase motility, lifespan, velocity and forward progression of spermatozoa of poor quality[1,2]. While it is generally true that non-motile spermatozoa are non-fertile, the converse that motile spermatozoa are able to fertilize is not necessarily true. There is a continuing controversy as to the value of caffeine in enhancing sperm motility and conception rates in the literature. Harrison[1] attempted artificial insemination using semen of men attending an infertility clinic with and without the addition of caffeine. He concluded that, although the motility of the spermatozoa was enhanced in each case, there was no increase in the pregnancy rate. Barkay[3], on the other hand, has found that the pregnancy rate may be significantly enhanced by the addition of caffeine to cryo-preserved human spermatozoa prior to insemination.

The zona-free hamster ova penetration test offers a tool by which the fertilization potential of sperm is assessed biologically by stimulating the last events in the fertilization process. It has been shown that the test is superior to routine seminal fluid analysis by its ability to clearly discriminate fertile from infertile men[4,5]. It has been the purpose of this work to assess the effect of caffeine on sperm penetration into zona-free hamster ova, and thus clarify the significance of exogenous addition of caffeine to fresh and freeze–thawed semen.

MATERIAL AND METHODS

In order to assess the effect of caffeine on spermatozoal ability to penetrate into zona-free hamster ova two types of sperm were utilized: (1) fresh semen samples submitted for routine analysis to our male infertility clinic and (2) cryopreserved semen samples for use in our AID programme. In cryopreservation 10% glycerol (v/v) is used as a protective medium. Samples are frozen in liquid nitrogen at $-196\,°C$. Samples were allowed to thaw at room temperature.

Each sample of either fresh or freeze–thawed semen was divided into two equal parts. To one half, caffeine was added to give a final concentration of 7 mmol/l, to the other, which served as control, an equal volume of normal saline was added.

The effect of caffeine on sperm penetration was evaluated after its addition at two different times: (1) immediately after liquefaction of either fresh or freeze–thawed sperm and (2) shortly before insemination of the zona-free hamster ova by sperm, washed and capacitated as described in the human hamster zona-free egg penetration test[4,5].

Four groups were studied (Table 1).

Table 1   Type of semen and timing of caffeine addition in the different groups studied

Group	Semen	No. of samples	Addition of caffeine (mmol/l)	Addition of NaCl (control)
I	fresh	6	after liquefaction	after liquefaction
II	freeze–thawed	6	after thawing	after thawing
III	fresh	6	before insemination	before insemination
IV	freeze–thawed	6	before insemination	before insemination

To evaluate any possible relationship between spermatozoal motility and penetration rates motility was assessed 30 minutes after the addition of either caffeine or saline, using the Makler Chamber.

Statistical analyses were performed with Student's paired t-test.

RESULTS

Mean changes in motility rates and penetration rates of 24 semen samples incubated with caffeine in comparison to control samples are shown in Table 2.

Table 2 The effect of caffeine on sperm motility and sperm penetration rates

	Motility (%)				Penetration (%)			
Group	Control (mean ± SE)	Caffeine (mean ± SE)	Increase[a] (%)	p value[b]	Control (mean ± SE)	Caffeine (mean ± SE)	Increase[a] (%)	p value[b]
I	33.8±4.1	45 ±5.1	33	0.002	20.7±10.3	20.6± 8.2	0	NS
II	33.3±5.0	42.5±5.0	28	0.01	42.7±13.8	39 ±14.3	−9	NS
III	27.3±4.7	31.7±3.8	16	0.05	24.7±11.9	24.8±10.5	0	NS
IV	30.5±7.2	35.7±7.5	17	0.05	35.5±12.0	36.5±13.9	3	NS
Overall	31.2±2.6	38.7±2.8	24	0.0001	30.9± 5.9	29.4± 5.9	−5	NS

$^a \dfrac{\text{Caffeine} - \text{control}}{\text{control}} \times 100$

[b] Paired t-test

NS – not significant

39

A mean overall increase of 24% in motility rates is noted with caffeine ($p < 0.0001$). The enhancing effect of caffeine upon motility is more pronounced when added to whole semen (group I and group II) than if added shortly before insemination – after sperm washing and incubation (group III and group IV). In contrast to the significant enhancing effect of caffeine on spermatozoal motility there is virtually no effect at all on penetration rates into zona-free hamster ova (Table 2).

COMMENTS

Caffeine is an inhibitor of cyclic nucleotide phosphodiesterases, enzymes also involved in spermatozoal glycolysis. It increases intracellular levels of cyclic AMP within minutes after addition to a semen specimen, and thus probably affects motility, by phosphorylation, of a protein essential to the regulation of spermatozoal motility[1].

Routine semen evaluation, which assesses total sperm count, sperm density, semen volume, rate and grade of spermatozoal progression and sperm morphology, gives some information of the fertility potential of a certain male, but the correlation of any parameter with fertility is far from good. The test that offers, to date, the best correlation with fertility potential is the zona-free hamster ova penetration assay[5]. Our study incorporating this assay, indicates that despite a significant increase in motility of spermatozoa with the addition of caffeine, no change is noted in penetration rates into zona-free hamster ova.

References

1. Harrison, R. F. (1978). Insemination of husband's semen with and without the addition of caffeine. *Fertil. Steril.*, **29**, 532
2. Amelar, R. D., Dubin, L. and Schoenfeld, C. Y. (1980). Sperm motility. *Fertil. Steril.*, **34**, 197
3. Barkay, J. (1979). Cryopreservation of semen and artificial insemination. Presented at the *First Pan-American Conference on Andrology*, March 13–16, Toronto
4. Rogers, B. J., Van Campen, H., Veno, M., Lambert, H., Bronson, K. and Hale, R. (1979). Analysis of human spermatozoal fertilizing ability using zona free ova. *Fertil. Steril.*, **32**, 64
5. Margalioth, E. J., Laufer, N., Navot, D., Voss, R. and Schenker, J. G. (1983). Reduced fertilization ability of zona-free hamster ova by spermatozoa from male partners of normal infertile couples. *Arch. Androl.*, **10**, 67

9
The variability and clinical value of a heterologous ovum penetration test

P. L. MATSON, J. P. PRYOR, R. CURSON and W. P. COLLINS

INTRODUCTION

The use of semen analysis, for the assessment of reproductive potential in the male partner of an infertile couple, usually gives considerable intra- and inter-man variation in the results, even under well-defined conditions. Notwithstanding this limitation, there have been reports in which an attempt has been made to relate fertility to the density of the spermatozoa[1], their progressive motility and the percentage with normal morphology[2]. The main conclusion from these studies, however, is that azoospermia is the only reliable index of infertility from a spermiogram. An alternative approach has developed from the observation that human spermatozoa are capable of penetrating zona-free hamster ova after an *in vitro* incubation, which is probably associated with capacitation[3]. Also, results from studies on the clinical application of the test have shown impaired penetration to be related to some forms of infertility[4].

The initial aim of this study was to apply the test to a cross-section of male patients attending an infertility clinic, to determine the proportion of negative results and the range of positive values. In addition, a second longitudinal study was undertaken to assess the within-man variation in (1) a fertile volunteer; and (2) a group of patients.

MATERIALS AND METHODS

Subjects and semen

The patients studied were the male partners of couples attending the infertility clinic at King's College Hospital, who had previously been found to have

41

normal spermiograms (i.e. semen volume 2–6 ml; sperm density $20–250 \times 10^6 \, ml^{-1}$; > 40% motile spermatozoa; > 60% normal morphological forms). The volunteer for the longitudinal study was aged 26 years at the start and of proven fertility. All semen specimens were collected (following 2 days sexual abstinence) into wide-mouthed, sterile, propylene universal containers, and processed within 2 h of collection.

Collection and examination of ova

Adult female golden hamsters (*Mesocricetus auratus*) were induced to super-ovulate by an intraperitoneal injection of 40 iu pregnant mares serum gonadotrophin (PMSG; Intervet Laboratories Ltd., Cambridge, UK), given irrespective of the day of the oestrous cycle, followed 72 h later by 25 iu of human chorionic gonadotrophin (Pregnyl; Organon Laboratories Ltd., Morden, Surrey, UK). The preparation of the spermatozoa, treatment of ova with enzymes, and co-culture of spermatozoa with zona-free eggs have been

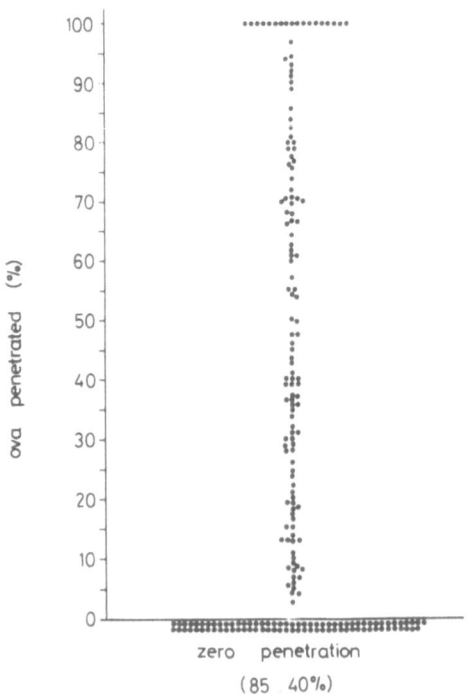

Figure 1   Penetration of zona-free hamster ova by spermatozoa from male partners ($n = 213$) of infertile couples

reported previously[4]. Suspensions of spermatozoa were adjusted to a constant density of $5 \times 10^6 \, ml^{-1}$. The end-point of the test was determined by examining compressed ova using Nomarski optics, and the definitive evidence of penetration was taken to be a spermatozoon, with a swollen head connected to the tail, inside the egg vitellus. The results were expressed as the percentage of the total number of ova (20–25 per patient) that had been penetrated, with the penetration of no ova being regarded as a negative result.

RESULTS AND DISCUSSION

Cross-sectional study

The results of the first test performed on samples from 213 patients are shown in Figure 1. It may be seen that the penetration rates ranged from 0 to 100%. Spermatozoa from 40% (85 out of 213) of subjects failed to penetrate any ova, and the wide range of positive values is similar to that reported elsewhere[5]. The results are not surprising since the couples presented with a variety of problems. However, the main feature of clinical significance is the proportion of negative results[6], which is in contrast with results obtained from groups of fertile men[7].

Longitudinal study

The 53 results obtained from a fertile volunteer over a period of 2 years are shown in Figure 2. It may be seen that the test results ranged from 12 to 100%. This finding is similar to that in our previous study[4], and those of other workers[8], although less variability has been reported elsewhere[9]. Also, a similar degree of variability has been shown to be associated with different periods of sexual abstinence by the subject prior to the collection of the semen specimen, and a varied exposure of the spermatozoa to seminal plasma after the sample has been produced[10]. Notwithstanding these limitations, it should be emphasized that the results in the present study were invariably positive, i.e. a number of ova were always penetrated.

Fifty three patients were tested two or more times. Consistently positive or negative (i.e. zero penetration) results were given by 24 and 22 men, respectively. Conflicting results were obtained in seven patients, but a closer examination of the data revealed that only one gave distinctly different results on successive occasions (0%, 64%, 36%). This patient was found to have evidence of a genital tract infection (routine semen analysis showed 82 round cells/high-power field) and he was treated with antibiotics. At the second and third tests there were 9 and 17 round cells/high-power field respectively, and the penetration rates were greatly improved. Such an association between

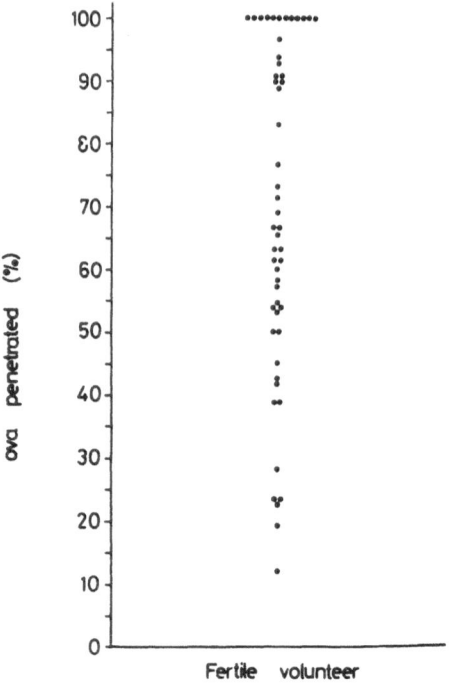

Figure 2 Penetration of zona-free hamster ova by spermatozoa from ejaculates ($n=52$) obtained from a healthy, fertile volunteer over a 2-year period

pyospermia and poor penetration of ova has been reported previously[11]. Spermatozoa from the other six patients all gave negative/low ova penetration rates (0%, 6%; 0%, 5%; 8%, 0%; 4%, 0%; 0%, 4%, 0%; 4%, 0%, 0%). This inconsistency may well reflect only a small population of spermatozoa in the incubation droplet which are capable of successfully interacting with the zona-free ova, which might be detected with a greater number of ova per test.

CONCLUSIONS

The use of zona-free hamster ova offers an *in vitro* test of male fertility, and provides a means of identifying patients whose spermatozoa are incapable of successfully interacting with ova. The test gave consistent results (i.e. positive or negative) in the majority of men re-tested, despite large inter- and intra-man variation in the positive values obtained.

References

1. Van Zyl, J. A., Menkveld, R., Refif, A. E. and Niekirk, W. A. (1976). Oligozospermia. In Hafez, E. S. E. (ed.) *Human Semen and Fertility Regulation in Men.* pp. 363–9. (St. Louis: C. V. Mosby)
2. Eliasson, R. (1977). Semen analysis and laboratory workup. In Cockett, A. T. K. and Urry, R. L. (eds.) *Male Infertility.* pp. 169–88. (New York: Grune and Stratton)
3. Yanagamachi, R., Yanagamachi, H. and Rogers, B. J. (1976). The use of zona-free animal ova as a test system for the assessment of the fertilizing capacity of human spermatozoa. *Biol. Reprod.*, **15**, 471
4. Tyler, J. P. P., Pryor, J. P. and Collins, W. P. (1981). Heterologous ovum penetration by human spermatozoa. *J. Reprod. Fertil.*, **63**, 499
5. Hammond, M. G., Sloan, C. S. and Hall, J. L. (1982). Application of interspecies *in vitro* fertilization in the initial assessment of the infertile couple. *Am. J. Obstet. Gynecol.*, **142**, 340
6. Matson, P. L., Pryor, J. P. and Collins, W. P. (1982). Heterologous ova penetration by human spermatozoa. Presented at the *Annual Conference of the Society for the Study of Fertility,* July 13–16, Nottingham
7. Zausner-Guelman, B., Blasco, L. and Wolf, D. P. (1981). Zona-free hamster eggs and human sperm penetration capacity: a comparative study of proven fertile donors and infertile patients. *Fertil. Steril.*, **36**, 771
8. Binor, Z., Sokoloski, J. E. and Wolf, D. P. (1980). Penetration of the zona-free hamster egg by human sperm. *Fertil. Steril.*, **33**, 321
9. Cohen, J., Weber, R. F. A., van der Vijver, J. C. M. and Zeilmaker, G. H. (1982). *In vitro* fertilizing capacity of human spermatozoa with the use of zona-free hamster ova: interassay variation and prognostic value. *Fertil. Steril.*, **37**, 565
10. Rogers, B. J., Perreault, S. D., Bentwood, B. J., McCorville, C., Hale, R. W. and Soderdahl, D. W. (1983). Variability in the human-hamster *in vitro* assay for fertility evaluation. *Fertil. Steril.*, **39**, 204
11. Berger, R. E., Karp, L. E., Williamson, R. A., Koehler, J., Moore, D. E. and Holmes, K. K. (1982). The relationship of pyospermia and seminal fluid bacteriology to sperm function as reflected in the sperm penetration assay. *Fertil. Steril.*, **37**, 557

10
Laser-induced stimulation of sperm motility *in vitro*

H. SATO, M. LANDTHALER, D. HAINA and W.-B. SCHILL

INTRODUCTION

Laser light of low energy density brings about stimulating effects on the growth of *E. coli*, the synthesis of haemoglobin and synthesis of collagen in wounds[1]. To study the laser effect on a living cell system, vital spermatozoa were used as a biological model. The aim of the present study was to prove if sperm motility and velocity are stimulated by laser radiation of low power density.

MATERIALS AND METHODS

Semen samples were obtained by masturbation from normal subjects and from patients with infertility disorders. A total of 15 ejaculates were used, and for each experiment 0.5 ml aliquots were transferred into seven microcuvettes. These aliquots were irradiated with krypton laser red light ($\lambda = 647$ nm) at different dosages. After 30 minutes incubation at room temperature, total sperm motility and velocity were measured by the multiple exposure photography method[2].

To eliminate the thermal effect of laser light, temperatures of the aliquots were measured before and after irradiation with an electric thermometer. The data obtained were expressed as mean value $\pm$ SE and assessed by paired student's *t*-test.

RESULTS

Total sperm motility increased after laser irradiation at 4 J/cm² ($p < 0.05$),

47

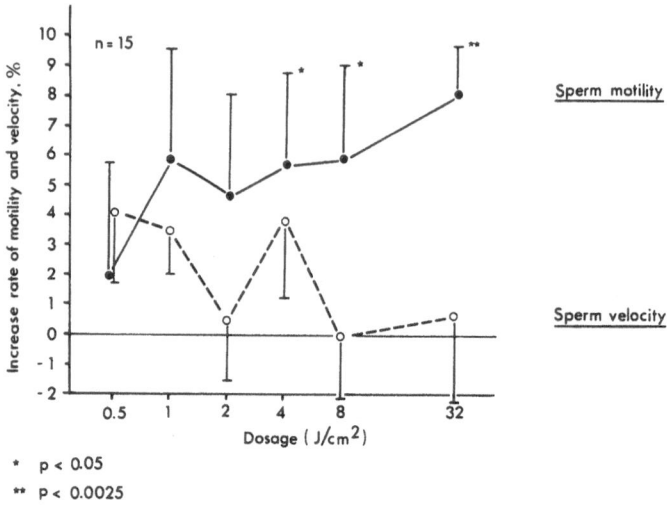

* p < 0.05
** p < 0.0025

Figure 1 Relative change of sperm motility and velocity with different dosage of laser light

$8 J/cm^2$ ($p<0.05$) and $32 J/cm^2$ ($p<0.0025$) respectively, with respect to control, non-irradiated spermatozoa (Figure 1). The most effective dosage, leading to an increase of the total sperm motility, was $32 J/cm^2$ and the mean increase rate was $8.1\% \pm 1.7\%$. At the dosage of $1.0 J/cm^2$, sperm motility increased by $5.7\% \pm 3.6\%$, but this was not significant due to great variations.

No influence on sperm velocity was demonstrated after laser irradiation. Temperature difference before and after laser irradiation was maximum at $32 J/cm^2$ and was within $0.3 °C$.

DISCUSSION

The stimulating effect of laser light on sperm motility is clearly demonstrated in this experiment. The increase rate of sperm motility was 8.1% at $32 J/cm^2$. Since stimulating effects of laser light have been proved only at low energy density[1], higher energy laser light than $32 J/cm^2$ was not used in this experiment.

Sperm motility is also stimulated by caffeine and kallikrein[3]. The increased rate of motility due to these agents is given as $50-80\%$ according to the literature. The stimulating effect of laser light on sperm motility is low compared to these substances.

Makler et al.[4] reported that during the phase of heating from room temperature to $37 °C$, sperm velocity increased, but no significant change in percentage

48

of motility was demonstrated. Therefore, the effect of laser light on motility is not due to a thermal effect but may be due to photobiological processes.

Sperm velocity was not stimulated by laser light. This observation may suggest that it does not influence moving spermatozoa, but probably stimulates non-motile live spermatozoa.

ACKNOWLEDGEMENT

This research was supported by grants of the Deutsche Forschungsgemein-schaft Schi 86/7–4 and Sonderforschungsbereich No. 0207 LP-20; and a fellowship (H.S.) from the Alexander von Humboldt Foundation, Bonn.

References

1. Schreiber, G. and Staupendahl, G. (1975). Laser in der Dermatologie. *Deutsch. Gesundh. Wes.*, **30**, 570
2. Makler, A. (1978). A new multiple exposure photography method for objective sperm motility determination. *Fertil. Steril.*, **30**, 192
3. Schill, W.-B. (1975). Caffeine- and kallikrein induced stimulation of human sperm motility: a comparative study. *Andrologia*, **7**, 229
4. Makler, A. *et al.* (1981). Factors affecting sperm motility VIII, *Int. J. Androl.*, **4**, 559

11

Time-sequential observation on human sperm penetration into zona pellucida-free hamster oocytes by scanning electron microscopy

A. TSUIKI, M. SUZUKI, K. HOSHI, K. KYONO, H. IMAIZUMI and H. HOSHIAI

INTRODUCTION

We have made time sequential observations on sperm–egg interactions in the zona-free hamster eggs–human sperm system with the scanning electron microscope.

Such studies serve the two-fold purpose of gaining information on the mechanism of sperm entry into oocytes, and determining if this heterologous system behaves similarly to the homologous system.

The establishment of similarities in the morphology of fertilization will help to validate this system as a reasonable model of the normal physiological pathway[1].

MATERIALS AND METHODS

Semen samples were obtained from fertile donors, and a sperm suspension ($5-10 \times 10^6$ motile sperm/ml) was placed under mineral oil in a plastic petri-dish.

After sperm preincubation, the zona pellucida-free hamster eggs were introduced into this suspension. At various times after incubation some eggs were removed for electron microscope processing, others were examined with

51

phase-contrast microscopy, and classified as 'fertilized' when swollen sperm heads and sperm midpiece were present in the ooplasm.

RESULTS

Most spermatozoa appear to be attached to the egg surface at a shallow angle or virtually parallel (Figure 1). Few spermatozoa are oriented to the surface perpendicularly. There was a tendency for greater sperm numbers to be attached at the egg surface as the sperm preincubation time was prolonged. Although the large majority of spermatozoa observed on the oocyte surface was acrosome-reacted, we occasionally observed spermatozoa with a partially

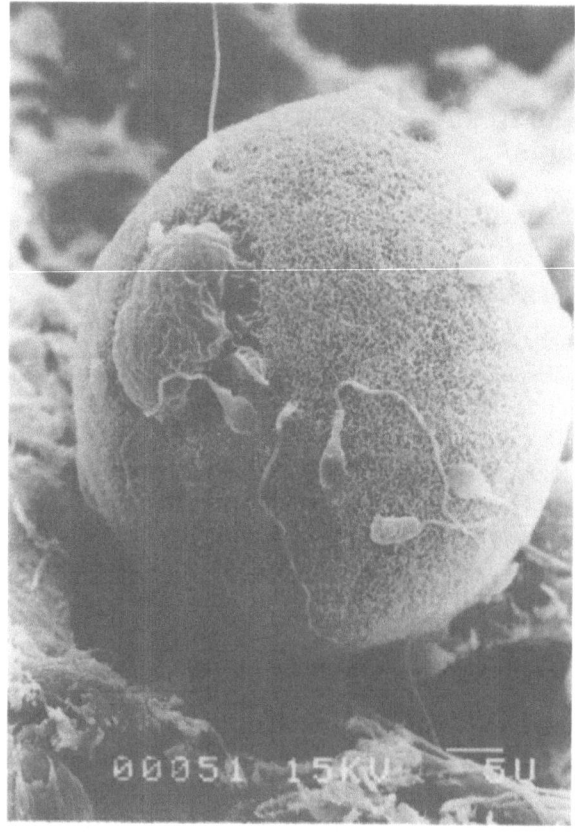

Figure 1 Human sperm bound to the surface of a zona pellucida free hamster oocyte ($\times 1050$)

intact acrosome on the oocyte surface (Figure 2). In acrosome-reacted spermatozoa, a ridge exists at the leading edge of the equatorial segments.

Many microvilli are shown to participate in sperm–egg interaction. After the initial contact with the surface of the ovum, the sperm head is trapped by elongated microvilli. Initially, microvilli appeared to grasp and immobilize the anterior tip of the sperm. But with the process of gamete interaction microvilli appears to trap the sperm head at the region of equatorial segment (Figure 3), leading to the covering of the ovum with cytoplasmic protrusions (Figure 4). Such spermatozoa may be partially submerged into ooplasm. Scanning electron micrography shows that the post-acrosomal region is first incorporated into the ooplasm. The anterior tip of the sperm head is the last portion to be incorporated.

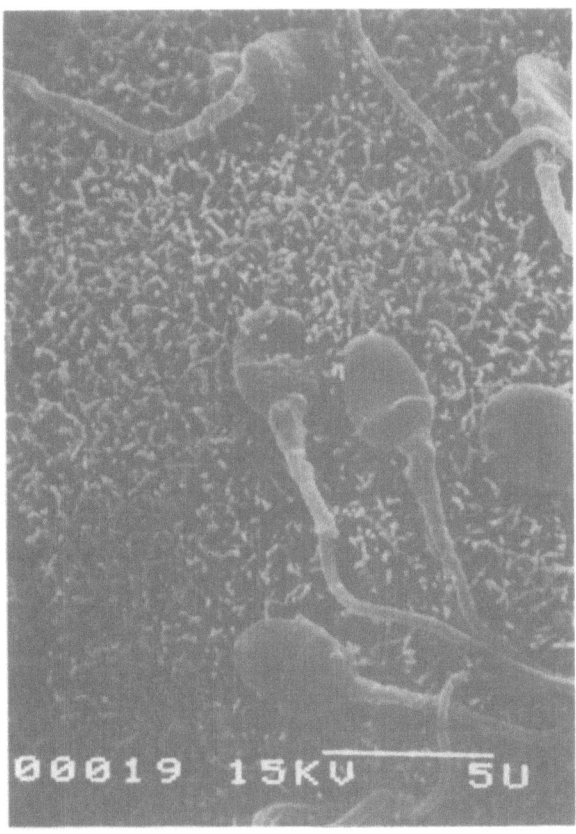

Figure 2 Most bound spermatozoa were acrosome-reacted. A ridge exists at the leading edge of the equatorial segment (×2450)

53

The microvilli of the oolenmal surface where sperm penetrated did not show major changes in size nor in appearance, and the so called 'incorporation cone' is not observed (Figure 5).

DISCUSSION

Our scanning electron micrographs illustrate that the microvillar portion of the oolenma greatly participated in this heterologous gamete interaction. With regard to sperm penetration into ovum this heterologous system behaves similarly to the homologous system.

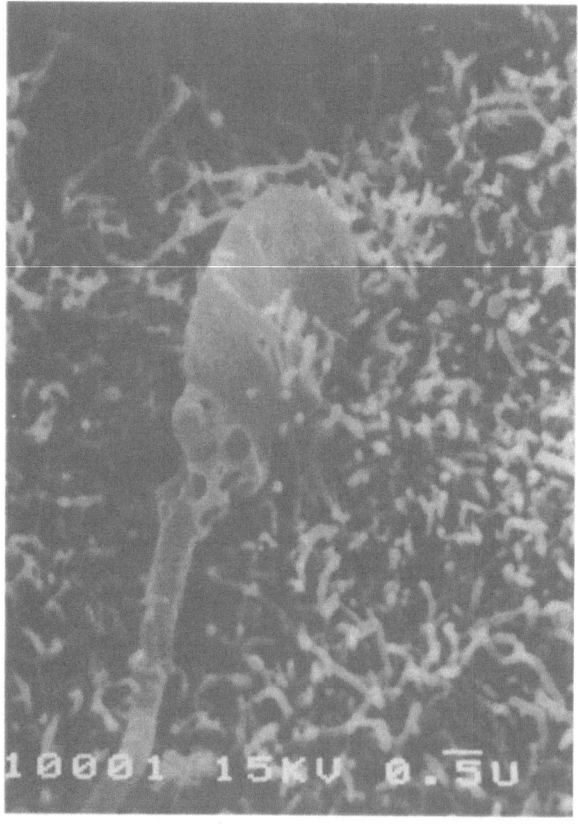

Figure 3 Microvilli were observed adjacent to the plasma membrane over the equatorial segment ($\times$ 4900)

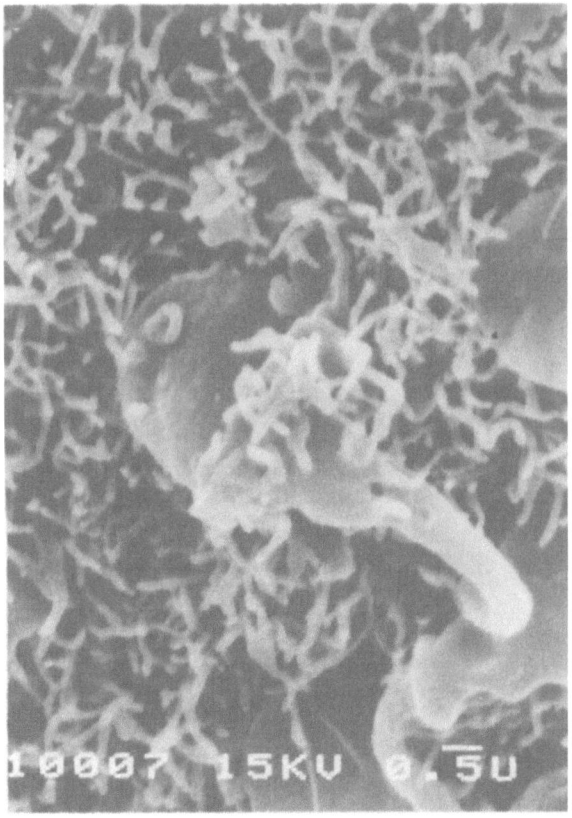

Figure 4   Equatorial segment was covered with cytoplasmic protrusions of the ovum (× 7000)

References

1. James, K. K., Ivan, D., Morton, A. S. and Dianne, S. (1982). Interaction of human sperm with zona-free hamster eggs. *A freeze–fracture study. Gamete Res.*, **6**, 371

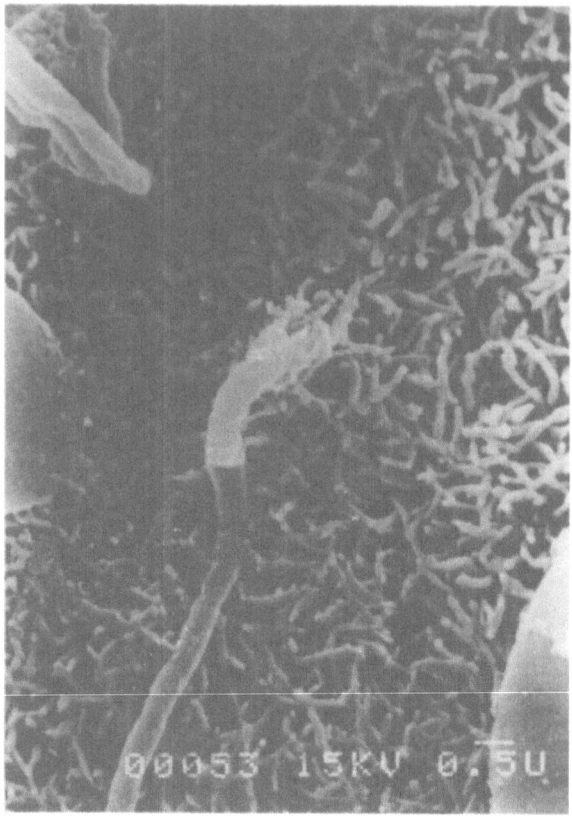

Figure 5 Oolemnal surface where sperm penetrated (×7000)

12
Analysis of various experimental conditions on the rate of human sperm penetration into zona-free hamster ova

E. J. MARGALIOTH, D. NAVOT, R. RABINOWITZ, N. LAUFER,
R. VOSS and J. G. SCHENKER

INTRODUCTION

Although routine microscopic sperm evaluation is, and will be, the primary tool for the assessment of human fertility potential it is fraught with many disadvantages: the most important is the indirectness of the various parameters. Semen volume, sperm number and concentration, sperm morphology and motility, all are criteria that correlate with fertility potential but neither prove nor disprove the actual fertilizing ability of spermatozoa. The human sperm penetration into zona-free hamster ova test comes closest to fulfilment of the need of a test assessing male fertility directly. The superiority of the sperm penetration test was demonstrated by Rogers and co-workers[1] and corroborated later by other groups[2,3,5].

Apart from its clinical application, this test has been utilized in the investigation of genetic, immunologic and biochemical aspects of sperm biology. Whilst the test is gaining wide acceptance, both in clinical use and basic research, the lack of a standardized methodology gives rise to a variety of modifications introduced by the different laboratories[1-4].

This work describes the effect of three parameters – source of serum albumin, its concentration, and sperm pre-incubation time – on the rate of human sperm penetration into zona-free hamster ova, and it presents an evaluation of two different methods of assessing penetration rate. By comparing these parameters, an attempt is made to define standard indices for the zona-free hamster ova penetration test.

MATERIALS AND METHODS

Semen samples were collected by masturbation into sterile containers after a period of sexual abstinence of at least 48 hours and allowed to liquefy for 60 minutes at room temperature. Following routine sperm analysis, the samples were poured into sterile 15 ml conical glass centrifuge tubes to determine their volume. Biggers, Whitten and Whittingham's medium (BWW)[6] containing 0.3% bovine serum albumin (BSA) was then added until a volume five times the original one was obtained. After two consecutive washings in BWW the third and final washing was performed and the sperm pellet was resuspended in 2 ml of medium containing different concentrations and sources of albumin:

(1) BWW containing 0.3% BSA,
(2) Modified BWW in which BSA concentration was increased to 3.5%,
(3) BWW with 0.3% human serum albumin (HSA), or
(4) Modified BWW with 3.5% HSA.

NaCl and bicarbonate concentrations were readjusted to maintain the same pH and osmolarity. The pellet was suspended in one of the above to a final sperm concentration of 10^7/ml. The sperm samples were incubated in 5% CO_2 at 37 °C for 2–18 h.

Ova were harvested from superovulated mature female hamsters. Egg preparation and stripping of the zona were performed by methods previously described[1,4]. Ten to 25 eggs were transferred into 0.1 ml sperm drops and incubated in 5% CO_2 in air, at 37 °C for 3 or 6 hours.

RESULTS

Table 1 demonstrates the superiority of HSA over BSA. Mean penetration rate using HSA was significantly higher than when using BSA (47% v. 28%, $p < 0.05$). Table 2 illustrates the advantage of higher concentrations of albumin both in terms of egg penetration rate and mean number of sperm per penetrated ovum (43.6% vs. 35%, 2.4% vs. 2.0; $p < 0.01$). Other experimental conditions were identical for all the tests conducted during this investigation.

To evaluate the extent to which pre-incubation affects sperm penetration, two equal aliquots obtained from the same semen sample were pre-incubated for 2 and 18 hours, respectively, after which both samples were mixed with ova and incubated for an additional 6 hours. The duration of pre-incubation did not influence penetration rates: 2 hour incubation yielded 33.5% penetration, compared to 33.3% after 18 hours.

Table 1 Comparison of sperm penetration rate using two sources of albumin[a]

	HSA 3.5%	BSA 3.5%
No. of samples	15	15
No. of ova examined	266	261
No. of penetrated ova	124	73
No. of penetrating sperm	214	98
Mean penetration (%)	47[b]	28[b]
Range of penetration	8–100	8–80
Mean number of sperm/penetrated ovum	1.7	1.7

[a] In all experiments, sperm pre-incubation lasted 18 hours and sperm–ova co-incubation continued for 3 hours
[b] $p < 0.05$

The penetration was assessed on 150 slides. Cover slips were pressed down on the eggs until the swollen sperm heads in the egg cytoplasm were clearly visible under a phase-contrast microscope at $\times 400$ magnification. The presence of a swollen sperm head of male pronucleus with a visible tail in the cytoplasm was considered positive penetration. The assessment of penetration was always done twice. Once for the freshly mounted ova, and later again after an overnight fixation with methanol:acetic acid, 3:1, and stained with 1% *aceto-lacmoid*. Examination of the living ova failed to detect 18% of the penetrated eggs and 25% of the penetrating sperm, failures which were subsequently revealed upon staining ($p < 0.01$).

DISCUSSION

Our results show that the penetration rate was increased in BWW medium containing 3.5% HSA as compared to 3.5% BSA or 0.3% HSA concentrations in the same medium. The importance of serum albumin as a major component

Table 2 Comparison of sperm penetration rate using two different concentrations of HSA[a]

	HSA 3.5%	HSA 0.3%
No. of samples	19	19
No. of ova examined	468	532
No. of penetrated ova	204	187
No. of penetrating sperm	485	368
Mean penetration (%)	43.6[b]	35[b]
Range of penetration	0–100	0–100
Mean number of sperm/penetrated ovum	2.4[b]	2.0[b]

[a] In all experiments, sperm pre-incubation lasted 18 hours and sperm–ova co-incubation continued for 3 hours
[b] $p < 0.01$

of BWW, or any other chemically defined medium for *in vitro* fertilization was shown by Yanagimachi[4]. Its main function in the media is to induce capacitation and acrosome reaction. Higher albumin concentrations may have a more pronounced enhancing effect on sperm capacitation, while the difference in penetration rates observed between HSA and BSA may be attributed to the relative higher purity of the HSA preparations. Pre-incubation induces capacitation and acrosome reaction of sperm. Although a gradual reduction in sperm motility after 18 hours of incubation was noted in our experiments, sperm penetration rate remained unaffected.

In conclusion, the experimental conditions tested with 3.5% HSA appeared optimal. Penetration rates did not differ with either 2 or 18 hours pre-incubation. The penetration rate of human spermatozoa into zona-free hamster ova should be assessed only after fixation and staining of the tested ova.

ACKNOWLEDGEMENT

This study was supported in part by a grant from the Joint Research Fund of the Hebrew University and Hadassah Hospital and the Samuel Pozzi Research Fund.

References

1. Rogers, B. J., Van Campen, H., Veno, M., Lambert, H., Bronson, R. and Hale, R. (1979). Analysis of human spermatozoal fertilizing ability using zona free ova. *Fertil. Steril.*, **32**, 664
2. Hall, J. L. (1981). Relationship between semen quality and human sperm penetration of zona free hamster ova. *Fertil. Steril.*, **35**, 457
3. Karp, L. E., Roger, A. W., Moore, D. E., Shy, K. K., Plymate, S. R. and Smith, W. D. (1981). Sperm penetation assay: useful test in evaluation of male fertility. *Obstet. Gynecol.*, **57**, 620
4. Yanagimachi, R., Yanagimachi, H. and Rogers, B. J. (1976). The use of zona free animal ova as a test system for the assessment of the fertilizing capacity of human spermatozoa. *Biol. Reprod.*, **15**, 471
5. Margalioth, E. J., Laufer, N., Navot, D., Voss, R. and Schenker, J. G. (1983). Reduced fertilization ability of zona-free hamster ova by spermatozoa from male partners of normal infertile couples. *Arch. Androl.*, **10**, 67
6. Biggers, J. D., Whitten, W. K. and Whittingham, D. F. (1971). The culture of mouse embryos in vitro. In Daniel, J. D. *Methods of Mammalian Embryology*, p. 101. (New York: Raven Press)

Section 2

Biochemistry of Gonadal Function

13
Levels of vitamin B_{12} and folic acid in seminal plasma from subjects with normal semen analysis and patients with idiopathic oligoasthenozoospermia

M. BRASSESCO, A. OLIVER, R. MORENO, F. MORER
and R. VILA

INTRODUCTION

Vitamin B_{12} and folic acid are indispensable coenzymes for a proper DNA synthesis during cellular mitosis. Tissues with a high metabolic index, e.g. testicular tissue, are more sensitive to a possible deficit of these coenzymes. Some pathologic conditions and longterm treatments with certain drugs can modify the levels or the tissue utilization of vitamin B_{12} and folic acid.

MATERIALS AND METHODS

Seminal plasma levels of vitamin B_{12} and folic acid were measured in 27 and 41 normal individuals, respectively, and in 40 subjects with different abnormalities in the semen analysis.

The following characteristics of semen analysis were considered normal: volume, 2–6 ml; sperm count about 80×10^6 per total ml of ejaculated semen; motility above 35% grade $+++$; morphology, at least 40% of the spermatozoa should be of normal size and shape, with the absence of inflammatory cells.

Commercial kits for radiometric analysis were used for vitamin B_{12} and folic acid assays in seminal plasma. These tests are based upon the competitive union with labelled vitamin (^{57}Co B$_{12}$ and ^{125}I-folate) and specific binding protein (porcine intrinsic factor and folate fixing factor of bovine milk).

The Student–Fisher's t-test, the Kolmogorov's test and the Mann–Whitney's test were used to analyse the data for statistical significance.

RESULTS

Seminal plasma levels of vitamin B$_{12}$ in a group of 27 individuals with normal semen analysis varied between 8 and 738 pmol/l (mean 191 pmol/l) (Table 1, Figure 1). There was a normal distribution of these values ($p < 0.01$) (Table 2).

All cases with different abnormalities in the semen analysis were grouped as a single class. Values for this group also followed a normal distribution ($p < 0.01$) (Table 2). There was a statistical significant difference between vitamin B$_{12}$ levels in this group and those in normal individuals ($p < 0.025$).

There were significant differences between the levels of vitamin B$_{12}$ in normal subjects (group I) and in patients with severe asthenozoospermia (group III) ($p < 0.05$). A comparison between normal individuals and patients

Table 1   Levels of vitamin B$_{12}$ in seminal plasma (pmol/l)

	Groups of patients	No. cases	Mean	Range
I	Normal	27	191	8–738
II	Moderate asthenozoospermia	14	144	0–528
III	Severe asthenozoospermia	6	40	0–124
IV	Severe oligoasthenozoospermia	9	107	0–265
V	Severe oligozoospermia	3	0	0

Table 2   Levels of vitamin B$_{12}$ in seminal plasma

Group of normal subjects:	
normal distribution*	$p < 0.01$
Group of patients:	
normal distribution*	$p < 0.01$

* Kolmogorov's test

Table 3   Levels of vitamin B$_{12}$ in seminal plasma. Comparison between groups

Group I/II	not significant
Group I/III	$p < 0.05$
Group I/IV	not significant
Group I/V	$p < 0.001$ (few data)

Mann–Whitney's test

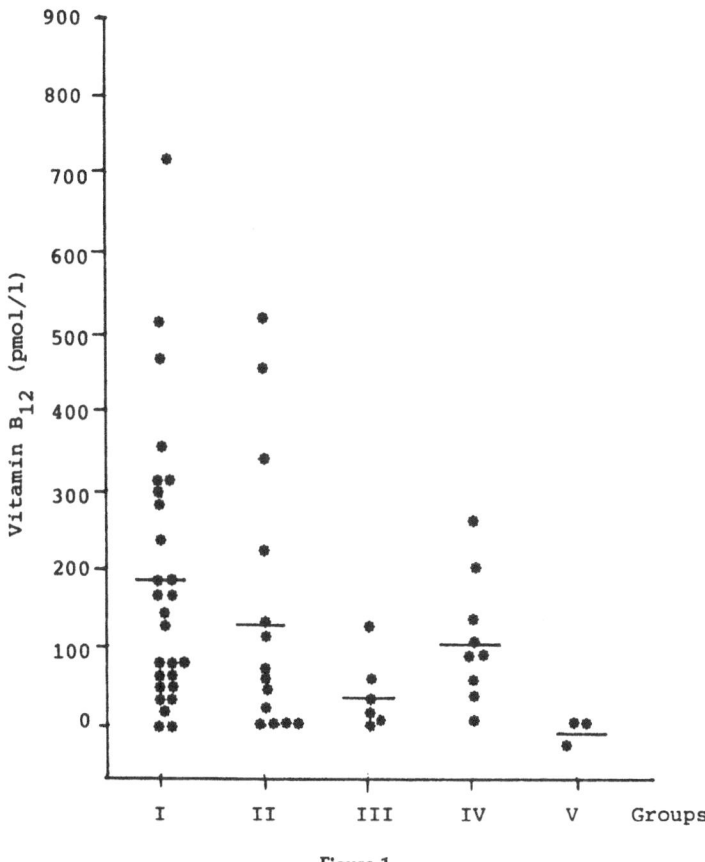

Figure 1

Table 4 Levels of folic acid in seminal plasma (nmol/l)

	Groups of patients	No. cases	Mean	Range
I	Normal	41	25	9–63
II	Moderate asthenozoospermia	13	27	18–48
III	Severe asthenozoospermia	10	30	18–48
IV	Severe oligoasthenozoospermia	13	22	11–32
V	Severe oligozoospermia	4	17	14–20

with severe oligozoospermia (group V) was also significant ($p < 0.001$) (Table 3).

Seminal plasma levels of folic acid in a series of 41 individuals with normal semen analysis varied from 9 to 63 nmol/l (mean 25 nmol/l) (Table 4, Figure 2). There was a normal distribution of these values ($p < 0.01$) (Table 5). How-

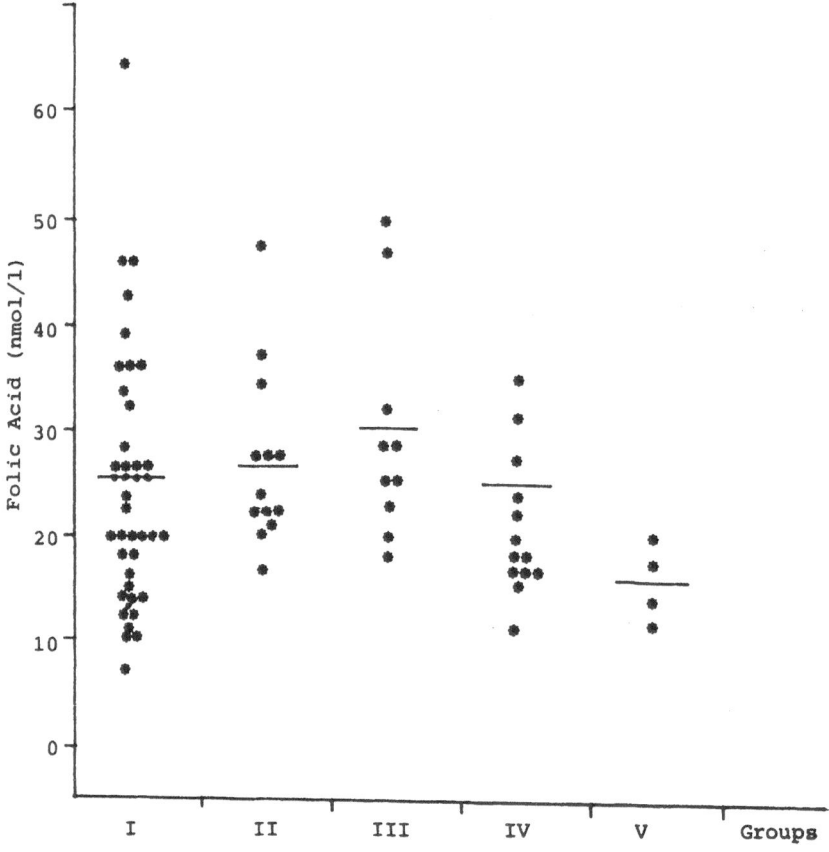

Figure 2 Levels of folic acid in seminal plasma

ever, an abnormal distribution law has been found when patients with different abnormalities in the semen analysis were grouped together (Table 5). Differences between this group and that of normal subjects were not statistically significant, although comparison between normal men and patients with severe oligozoospermia was significant ($p < 0.01$) (Table 6).

Table 5 Levels of folic acid in seminal plasma

Group of normal subjects: normal distribution*	$p < 0.01$
Group of patients: abnormal distribution*	n.s.

* Kolmogorov's test

Table 6 Levels of folic acid in seminal plasma. Comparison between groups

Group I/II	not significant
Group I/III	not significant
Group I/IV	not significant
Group I/V	$p<0.01$ (few data)

Mann–Whitney's test

DISCUSSION

According to these preliminary results measurement of seminal plasma levels of vitamin B$_{12}$ and folic acid could be a reliable method for the diagnosis of patients whose possible cause of infertility would be a deficit of these factors.

We have already detected extremely low levels of vitamin B$_{12}$ in several cases in the present series, all of them showing an abnormal semen analysis. In these circumstances the administration of vitamin B$_{12}$ and/or folic acid may offer the possibility of an effective therapy.

14
Functional role of relaxin in the human seminal fluid

F. KRASSNIGG, E. TÖPFER-PETERSEN, J. FRICK and W.-B. SCHILL

INTRODUCTION

Relaxin, a peptide hormone with structural homology to insulin, has long been regarded as a hormone of pregnant females having the function at parturition to relax the pelvic ligaments and to soften the cervix[1]. In certain animals relaxin also exerts a role in maintaining pregnancy by inhibiting uterine contractions[2]. So far relaxin has been characterized in extracts from ovaries of pregnant sows, rats, cows, rhesus monkeys and also from the placenta of the Sand Tiger Shark. In women relaxin is detectable in serum during pregnancy, and is synthesized in the ovaries and probably also in the placenta.

Little is known about relaxin in the male. Immunoreactivities could be demonstrated in extracts from the testes of armadillos and roosters, and also in boar testes. The human seminal plasma contains large amounts of relaxin-like immunoreactivity[3].

It was the aim of this study to identify that part of the reproductive system in the human male which is responsible for the synthesis of relaxin. Further to gain information about any regulatory function of relaxin on the angiotensin converting enzyme (ACE), since it is known that the structurally related hormone, insulin, inhibits the turnover of bradykinin by ACE. In addition, relaxin levels were determined in seminal plasma, and compared with other clinical parameters in groups of patients arranged according to their fertility potential.

MATERIALS AND METHODS

For the quantitative determination of relaxin, a heterologous radioimmuno-assay (RIA) with porcine relaxin as the standard according to a previously described method[4] was established. For qualitative registration a modified double antibody sandwich enzyme linked immunosorbent assay (ELISA) was used (publication in preparation). For the isolation of human relaxin, pooled seminal plasma was submitted to ion-exchange chromatography on carboxy-methylcellulose. The fraction containing relaxin immunoreactivity was further purified by affinity chromatography using immobilized IgG antibodies raised in rabbits against porcine relaxin. The final purification was achieved after gel-filtration on Sephadex G 50 by reverse phase chromatography. For the production of specific antibodies against human relaxin, isolated from seminal plasma, a mouse hybridoma cell line was established. Before the vaccination, relaxin was covalently bound to modified carrier proteins as described elsewhere[5]. Tissue extracts from human testes, prostate, epididymis and ovaries were prepared with equal amounts (w/v) of saline. For immuno-cytochemistry, prostatic tissue was serially sectioned and stained. The controls included male rabbit serum controls and reagent omission controls. ACE-activity was determined according to Cushman and Cheung[6]. For sperm motility studies each specimen was examined for total sperm count, morphologic characterization, total and progressive motility and chemical parameters. Only semen specimens with good initial motility were used after washing with Tyrode's solution. All samples used were from patients seeking advice for fertility disorders.

RESULTS

The seminal plasma relaxin levels determined with the heterologous RIA using porcine relaxin as standard were in patients with normozoospermia 7.3 ± 1.2 ng/ml ($n = 39$), in patients with oligozoospermia 6.32 ± 1.2 ng/ml ($n = 46$) and in patients with kryptozoospermia 6.2 ± 2.9 ng/ml ($n = 10$). In split-ejaculates ($n = 12$) the detectable relaxin amounts in the first fraction containing mainly the prostatic, testicular and epididymal secretions were significantly higher (2.1 ± 0.8 ng/ml) compared to the second fraction (0.45 ± 0.16 ng/ml) representing the seminal vesicle secretions. In patients suffering from Klinefelter's syndrome ($n = 13$) relaxin levels were 8.1 ± 1.8 ng/ml. No statistically significant correlation with the serum concentrations of LH, FSH and testosterone was detectable. No relaxin activity was detected in serum samples from men. In preliminary investigations no significant influence of porcine relaxin (10.0 ng/ml) on the motility of washed human spermatozoa was observed during an incubation period of 80 minutes at 37 °C.

The relaxin levels in extracts from human testes, epididymes, prostate glands and ovaries, determined with the ELISA technique showed, in the male, the highest levels in extracts from the prostatic gland. For immunocyto-chemical localization of the tissue that is responsible for the synthesis of relaxin in the male reproduction tract anti-porcine relaxin antibodies raised in rabbits were used. Subsequent treatment of prostatic tissue sections with anti-rabbit IgG–FITC conjugates (diluted 1/80 with PBS) resulted in positive staining of the secretory epithelium of the prostatic gland. The ACE-activity of the seminal plasma was not inhibited by porcine relaxin, applied in amounts ranging from 1 to 10 ng/ml, when the synthetic substrate N-α-Hippuryl-L-his-L-leu was used.

DISCUSSION

Relaxin-like immunoreactivity, expressed in our heterologous RIA as porcine relaxin-like equivalents, was detectable in all investigated human semen samples. However, in sera of male subjects relaxin could not be demonstrated, indicating that in men only the reproductive tract is responsible for the synthesis. In split-ejaculates the first fraction always showed significantly higher concentrations of the hormone, exhibiting the likely prostatic origin of relaxin. The immunocytochemical staining of human prostatic tissue sections demonstrates clearly the presence of relaxin-like immunoreactivity in the secretory epithelium. This finding supports the view that in the male relaxin is predominantly a product of the prostatic gland. This corresponds with similar results from other investigators[7].

There is only scanty information about the functional role of relaxin in the male reproduction tract. Any influence of relaxin on sperm motility[8] is however, according to our preliminary results, still speculative. The influence of porcine relaxin on the activity of the angiotensin converting enzyme (EC 3.4.15.1) present in seminal plasma was not detectable when a synthetic substrate, replacing the naturally used angiotensin I, was applied. However, a possible effect of relaxin on the kinin-inactivating activity of ACE cannot be excluded. This is in accordance with the fact that the structurally related hormone, insulin, inhibits the turnover of kinins (e.g. bradykinin) by ACE[9].

ACKNOWLEDGEMENT

This investigation was supported by the Deutsche Forschungsgemeinschaft, Sonderforschungsbereich 0207, Project No. LP 20.

References

1. Steinitz, B.G., Beach, V.L. and Kroc, R.L. (1959). The Physiology of Relaxin in Laboratory Animals. In Lloyd, C. (ed.) *Recent Progress in Endocrinology of Reproduction*. pp. 389–427 (New York: Academic Press)
2. Porter, D.G. and Downing, S. (1978). Evidence that a humoral factor possessing relaxin-like activity is responsible for uterine quiescence in the late pregnant rat. *J. Reprod. Fertil.*, **52**, 95
3. Loumaye, E., Decooman, S. and Thomas, K. (1980). Immunoreactive relaxin-like substance in human seminal plasma. *J. Clin. Endocrinol. Metab.*, **50**, 1142
4. O'Byrne, E.M. and Steinitz, B.G. (1976). Radioimmunoassay (RIA) of relaxin in serum of various species using an antiserum to porcine relaxin. *Proc. Soc. Exp. Biol. Med.*, **152**, 272
5. Krassnigg, F., v. Werder, K. and Bock, L. (1982). Isolation and characterization of relaxin from human placenta. *Fresenius Z. Anal. Chem.*, **311**, 359
6. Cushman, D.W. and Cheung, H.S. (1971). Spectrophotometric assay and properties of the angiotensin converting enzyme of rabbit lung. *Biochem. Pharmacol.*, **20**, 1637
7. Essig, M., Schoenfeld, C., D'Eletto, R., Amelar, R., Dublin, L., Steinitz, B.G., O'Byrne, E.M. and Weiss, G. (1982). Relaxin in human seminal plasma. In Steinitz, B.G., Schwabe, Ch. and Weiss, G. (eds.) *Relaxin: Structure, Function, and Evolution*. pp. 224–29 (New York: Ann. NY Acad. Sci., vol. 380)
8. Essig, M., Schoenfeld, C., Amelar, R.D., Dubin, L. and Weiss, G. (1982). Stimulation of human sperm motility by relaxin. *Fertil. Steril.*, **38**, 339
9. Erdös, E.G. (1979). Bradykinin, kallidin and kallikrein. In Eicher, O., Farah, A., Herken, H. and Welch, A.D. (eds), *Handbook of Experimental Pharmacology*. pp. 459 (Berlin, Heidelberg, New York: Springer)

15
Hyperprolactinaemia and abnormal seminal cytology

D. SULTAN SHERIFF

INTRODUCTION

Apart from its established role in lactation in females, there is a considerable body of evidence to suggest a role for prolactin (PRL) in the testis and the male accessory organs[1]. These data include the demonstration of binding sites, trophic effects, stimulation of steroidogenesis, stimulation of steroid-metabolizing enzymes and effects on spermatogenesis[2-6]. In normoprolactin-aemia, PRL has little or no effect by itself, but potentiates the effect of LH on steroidogenesis, and synergizes with testosterone in its effect on the prostate and seminal vesicles[4]. PRL modulates testicular function by a direct effect on the Leydig cells, on their ability to bind LH[3,7]. The apparent stimulation of FSH release by PRL may also contribute to its influence on testicular steroido-genesis[1]. In the ejaculate PRL stimulates the ATPase activity of human spermatozoa, thus influencing their motility and fertilizing capacity via effects on the energy metabolism[8-10]. In the case of hyperprolactinaemia, PRL seems to counteract gonadal steroidogenesis, metabolism of testosterone and sperm motility[11,17]. In the present study the effect of hyperprolactinaemia on seminal cytology of infertile patients is presented with a view to bring out the importance of PRL on spermatid differentiation.

MATERIALS AND METHODS

Among the different categories of infertile patients studied, eight patients with hyperprolactinaemia were taken for the present study. They were 25.00±5.00

years old. They were free from hepatic, renal or other endocrinological diseases that interfere with fertility. Of the eight patients studied, none had visual field defects or an enlarged sella turcica to suggest pituitary disease.

Semen samples were collected by masturbation into labelled glass containers after a period of 3–5 days abstinence. Sperm count, motility, morphology and volume were analysed by routine methods as described earlier[12]. The results were expressed as an average of three semen samples collected from each patient. Blood was collected from the patients between 8.30 and 10.30 a.m. under fasting conditions on three consecutive days. The sera were pooled and stored at $-30\,°C$. FSH, LH, PRL and T_4 were estimated by routine radioimmunoassay methods. Serum testosterone and oestradiol-17β levels were also estimated by specific radioimmunoassays. Interassay and intra-assay variation expressed as coefficients of variation were LH 15, 8; FSH 15, 8; PRL 15, 10; T 12, 10; E_2 15, 10; and T_4 12, 10, respectively. The levels of significance between the controls (normal volunteers of the age group 25.00 ± 6.50 years subjected to similar analyses) and the patients were calculated and expressed accordingly.

RESULTS

A marked reduction in sperm count ($p < 0.01$), sperm motility ($p < 0.01$) and an increase in abnormal forms of spermatozoa are observed in the patients. The abnormality was found to be due to abnormalities in tail structure (Table 1).

The levels of serum PRL and LH were elevated in the patients ($p < 0.01$) with normal levels of FSH, T_4 and oestradiol-17β. The levels of testosterone in the

Table 1 Seminal plasma composition of patients with hyperprolactinaemia*

Parameter	Controls	Patients	Statistical significance
Sperm count (million/ml)	65.00 ± 4.00	30.10 ± 5.00	$p < 0.01$
Sperm motility (% motility after 1 hour)	63.50 ± 4.50	40.00 ± 5.00	$p < 0.01$
Sperm morphology (%)	60.50 ± 4.00	45.00 ± 5.00	$p < 0.01$
Volume (ml)	3.00 ± 1.00	2.70 ± 1.25	NS

* Values are given as means $\pm$ SE of eight cases per group
NS = Not significant

74

patients were reduced when compared with the control group ($p < 0.05$) (Table 2).

DISCUSSION

Semen from infertile patients often contains a higher percentage of abnormal forms of spermatozoa than semen from fertile men[13]. The abnormality may either be due to abnormal structure or due to the presence of immature forms.

Such morphological abnormalities can be due to a variety of insults, including infection, testicular stress or hormonal imbalance[14]. The presence of many abnormal forms indicates impaired fertility. Such samples usually exhibit other abnormalities, including poor motility or low concentration. In fact there is an inverse correlation between abnormal forms and motility[15]. In the present study the patients had hormonal imbalance, as shown by the presence of elevated levels of PRL and LH and reduced levels of testosterone. The seminal analyses revealed the presence of abnormal forms of spermatozoa in the ejaculate with poor motility and lowered sperm counts. The abnormality of the spermatozoa was found to be due to tail defects. Kinking of tail structure with the presence of an enlarged cytoplasmic droplet was the major abnormality expressed in the spermatozoal structure. It is said that kinking of the tail probably occurs in the early stages of spermatid differentiation; the growing tail cannot stretch the cell membrane and then continues to develop within it. Such malformations can later interfere with sperm release from the Sertoli cells; when they do, an enlarged cytoplasmic droplet remains associated with the head or tail piece[14]. The presence of hyperprolactinaemia along with low testosterone levels may be the cause of such abnormalities associated with spermatid differentiation. It is also known that normal

Table 2 Endocrine profile of patients with hyperprolactinaemia*

Parameter	Controls	Patients	Statistical significance
Serum FSH (mIU ml^{-1})	13.05±2.50	20.10±2.75	NS
Serum LH (mIU ml^{-1})	12.05±4.50	50.00±4.75	$p < 0.01$
Serum PRL (ng ml^{-1})	8.75±0.45	35.00±1.00	$p < 0.01$
Serum testosterone (ng ml^{-1})	6.50±0.50	3.50±0.75	$p < 0.05$
Serum T$_4$ (μg ml^{-1})	6.00±3.00	6.50±3.25	NS
Serum E$_2$ (pg ml^{-1})	35.45±4.50	29.00±5.00	NS

* Values are means±SE of eight cases per group
NS = Not significant

testosterone levels are required for spermateleosis. Toth had shown the presence of such abnormal tail defects with enlarged cytoplasmic droplets in a single patient with a pituitary prolactin-secreting adenoma[16]. After surgical removal of the pituitary adenoma when the prolactin levels returned to normal, the patient's ejaculate had normal spermatozoa and good motility. This study seems to give a direct evidence for the participation of hyperprolactinaemia as a cause of inducing tail defects in the spermatozoal structure. In the present study the patients were not studied after bromocriptine therapy to implicate such an inhibitory role for PRL on testosterone-stimulated spermatid differentiation.

The increased levels of LH found in the patients may be due to an attempt to enhance androgen synthesis in the presence of partial androgen resistance. Segal et al.[17] seem to have felt that in humans such correlation or reciprocal relationship between gonadotrophins and PRL may not exist as observed in rats. But it does not rule out the possibility that a critical ratio between the gonadotrophins and PRL may be important for normal testosterone production. Any alteration may affect the testosterone production. It has recently been documented that chronically elevated levels of prolactin inhibits oestrogen production by suppressing aromatase activity in the ovary. PRL has also been reported to inhibit LH-stimulated androgen synthesis in the interstitial cells of the ovary, and this action appears to be exerted at the post-receptor level between cAMP production and pregnenolone formation[18]. In a similar manner, elevated levels of PRL may affect testosterone production thereby interfering with normal spermatid differentiation. Further studies are needed to elucidate the participation of PRL in the spermatogenic process in humans.

References

1. Bartke, A. (1980). Role of prolactin in reproduction in male mammals. *Fed. Proc.*, **39**, 2517
2. Charreau, E. H., Attramadal, A., Torjesen, P. A., Purvis, K., Calandra, R. and Hansson, V. (1977). Prolactin binding in rat testis. Specific receptors in interstitial cells. *Mol. Cell Endocrinol.*, **6**, 303
3. Aragona, C., Bohnet, H. G. and Friesen, H. G. (1977). Localization of prolactin binding in prostate and testis. The effect of serum prolactin concentration on testicular LH receptors. *Acta Endocrinol.*, **84**, 402
4. Negro-Vilar, A., Sadd, W. A. and McCann, S. M. (1977). Evidence for a role of prolactin in prostate and seminal vesicle growth in immature male rats. *Endocrinology*, **100**, 729
5. Hafiez, A. A., Lloyd, C. W. and Bartke, A. (1972). The role of prolactin in the regulation of testis function. The effects of prolactin and luteinizing hormone on the plasma levels of testosterone and androstenedione in hypophysectomized rats. *J. Endocrinol.*, **52**, 327
6. Musto, N., Hafiez, A. A. and Bartke, A. (1972). Prolactin increases 17β-hydroxysteroid dehydrogenase activity in the testis. *Endocrinology*, **91**, 1106
7. Purvis, K., Clausen, O. P. F., Olsen, A., Hing., E. and Hansson, V. (1979). Prolactin and leydig cell responsiveness to LH/HCG in the rat. *Arch. Androl.*, **3**, 219
8. Pedron, N. and Gimer, J. (1978). Effect of prolactin on the glycolytic metabolism of spermatozoa from infertile subjects. *Fertil. Steril.*, **29**, 428

9. Sheth, A. R., Gunjikar, A. N. and Shah, G. V. (1979). Effect of LH, prolactin and spermine on ATPase activity of human spermatozoa. *Andrologia*, **11**, 11
10. Shah, G. V., Desai, G. B. and Sheth, A. R. (1976). Effect of prolactin on metabolism of human spermatozoa. *Fertil. Steril.*, **27**, 1292
11. Hermanns, U. and Hafez, E. S. E. (1981). Prolactin and male reproductive physiology and physiopathology. In *Third World Congress of Human Reproduction*, Abstract volume, p. 124. (Berlin: International Academy of Reproductive Medicine)
12. Sultan Sheriff, D. (1983). Setting standard of male fertility. I. Semen analyses in 1500 men reporting for vasectomy. *Andrologia*, **15**, 687
13. Macleod, J. (1970). The significance of deviations in human sperm morphology in the human testis. *Adv. Exp. Med. Biol.*, **10**, 481
14. Alexander, N. J. (1982). Male evaluation and semen analyses. *Clin. Obstet. Gynecol.*, **25**, 463
15. Bartak, V. (1973). Sperm velocity and morphology in 1727 ejaculates with normal sperm count. *Int. J. Fertil.*, **18**, 116
16. Toth, A. (1981). Abnormal seminal cytology in a patient with prolactin-secreting pituitary adenoma. *Fertil. Steril.*, **36**, 818
17. Segal, S., Polistruk, W. Z. and Ben-David, M. (1976). Hyperprolactinaemic male infertility. *Fertil. Steril.*, **27**, 1425
18. Magoffin, D. A. and Ericksonn, G. F. (1982). Prolactin inhibition of leuteinizing hormone stimulated androgen synthesis in ovarian interstitial cells cultures in defined medium. Mechanism of action. *Endocrinology*, **111**, 2001

16
Serum FSH and spermatogenesis

J. H. NELSON, III, C. B. PASCHALL, III, W. BAIRD,
R. C. HARSH and M. A. DAVIS

ABSTRACT

Between August, 1981 and May, 1983 (21 months), 371 men were evaluated
for hypofertility. Data from semen analyses, testicular biopsies, and pooled
serum FSH (RIA) were analysed. FSH levels were investigated in 204 patients.
Bilateral testicular biopsies were performed on 104 patients. FSH was found to
be elevated in 18 of 30 patients (60%) who were azoospermic. 10 of 47 (47%) with
less than 20×10^6 ejaculated sperm, and 7 of 56 (12.5%) patients with
$20-50 \times 10^6$ sperm per ejaculate. No patients with more than 50×10^6 sperm
per ejaculate ($n = 74$) had an elevated FSH. Serum FSH does not seem
warranted in patients with more than 50×10^6 sperm per ejaculate (or 15×10^6
sperm per ml). Testicular biopsies, analysed by spermatid quantitation were
frequently very abnormal (25.6%) despite normal FSH levels, indicating a
failure of hypothalamic/pituitary response to hypospermatogenesis. Conversely, testicular biopsies were 'normal' in 36% of severely oligospermic men
($\leq 10 \times 10^6$ sperm/ejaculate) indicating potentially reconstructible lesions.

INTRODUCTION

The recognition of ductal obstruction as an important, potentially correctible
cause of male hypofertility has underscored the need for more precise means of
evaluating the functional integrity of the seminiferous epithelium. The fact
that obstruction can be partial and/or intermittent, yielding varying degrees of
oligozoospermia, has rendered the necessity of making this distinction even
more important. Elevation of serum FSH in the hypofertile man is well

recognized as a grim prognosticator with respect to treatment or ultimate pregnancy; however, no direct correlation exists between normal levels of that hormone and either semen quality as measured by sperm count or testicular histology.

Silber[1] has pointed out the importance of quantitative analysis of testicular biopsy specimens in the evaluation and prognostication of patients with oligozoospermia.

We studied the relationship between serum FSH, sperm count, and quantitative testicular biopsy in an attempt to further clarify the complex clinical classification and treatment of the hypofertile man.

MATERIALS AND METHOD

During the period from August, 1981–May, 1983, 371 men were evaluated for hypofertility. In addition to routine history and physical examination, contact scrotal thermography and detailed semen analysis with *in vitro* penetration testing (zona-free hamster ova, bovine cervical mucus) were performed. FSH, LH, testosterone, and prolactin (by RIA) were determined on pooled sera from three samples obtained over a 1 hour period on 224 patients. Bilateral testicular biopsies were performed on 104 patients for the following indications: (1) suspected obstruction (concurrently with scrotal exploration), (2) 'idiopathic' oligozoospermia, prior to treatment with clomiphene citrate, and (3) in conjunction with testicular vein ligation for varicocele.

Serum FSH values from 207 patients were considered for analysis (same laboratory). Testicular biopsy material from one hospital (74 cases) where pathologists routinely performed quantitative analysis by the method of Silber was included. In brief, tissue was sharply excised, fixed in Bouin's solution, and thinly sectioned. Mature spermatids were counted in a minimum of five seminiferous tubules and averages reported from each testis, and the mean of both.

Sperm counts on from two to three semen samples (minimum 3 week interval with usual abstinence period) were obtained and both sperm density (sperm/ml) and sperm total (volume × density) were averaged.

RESULTS

Data from 74 patients without ductal obstruction are listed in Table 1. No significant difference was seen in spermatid counts between right and left biopsies. Sperm density and sperm total, as expected, showed a high correlation ($r=0.92$). Serum FSH was elevated in 18 of 30 (60%) azoospermic patients and in a significant number of severely oligozoospermic patients (Figures 1 and 2) up to 15 million sperm/ml or 50 million sperm per ejaculate. Beyond

Table 1 Serum FSH, testicular biopsy, and semen analysis data in 74 patients without ductal obstruction

FSH	– 8.00±6.9	MIU/ml
Bx-Lt.	– 11.80±9.5	Spermatids/Tubule
Bx-Rt.	– 10.90±8.1	Spermatids/Tubule
Bx-Rt.+Lt.	– 11.20±7.9	Spermatids/Tubule
Sperm density	– 17.30±22.3	Sperm/ml
Sperm total	– 56.20±60.0	Sperm/Ejaculate mean±SD

those levels no elevated FSH assays were found (both significant, $p < 0.001$ by χ^2 analysis).

In 63 patients without ductal obstruction, mean spermatid count (L and R) was compared to both sperm density and total sperm per ejaculate with only fair correlation ($r = 0.42$, $r = 0.31$) (Figures 3 and 4).

Spermatid counts were, as expected, often quite abnormal despite normal FSH (Table 2) with 10 patients (25.6%) having levels of spermatogenesis at or below 1 SD from the mean of 7.9 spermatids/tubule.

In men with severe oligozoospermia ($\leq 10 \times 10^6$ sperm/ejaculate) but normal FSH levels, nine (36%) had spermatid counts at or above the mean for the non-obstructed group (11.2 spermatids/tubule) (Table 3) indicating a probable obstructive aetiology. In fact, of these nine patients, seven were documented

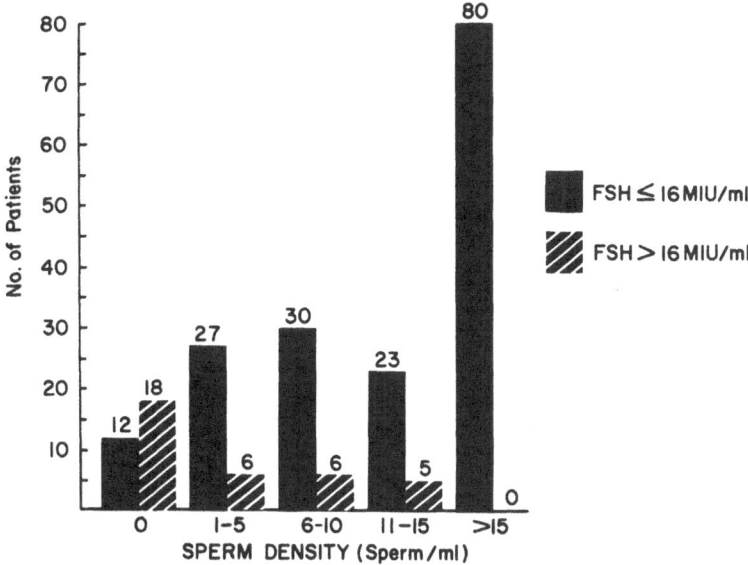

Figure 1 Serum FSH and sperm count as sperm/ml in 207 hypofertile men

81

to have an obstruction as follows: three ejaculatory duct obstruction, three epididymal obstruction, and one partial Wolffian duct agenesis.

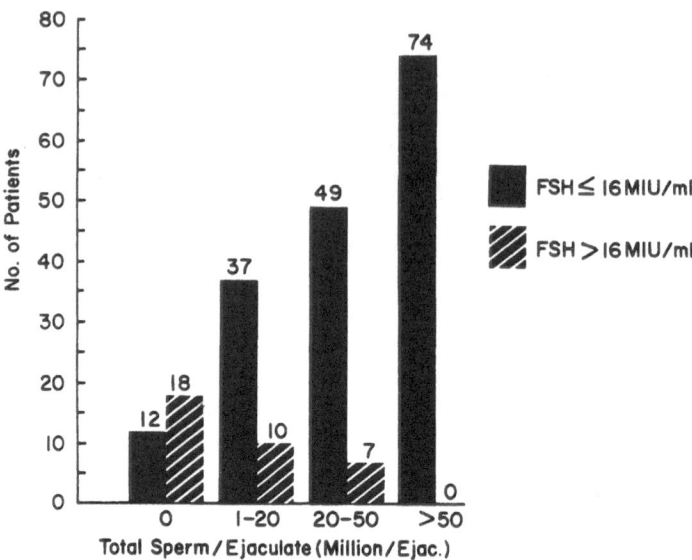

Figure 2   Serum FSH and sperm count as sperm/ejaculate in 207 hypofertile men

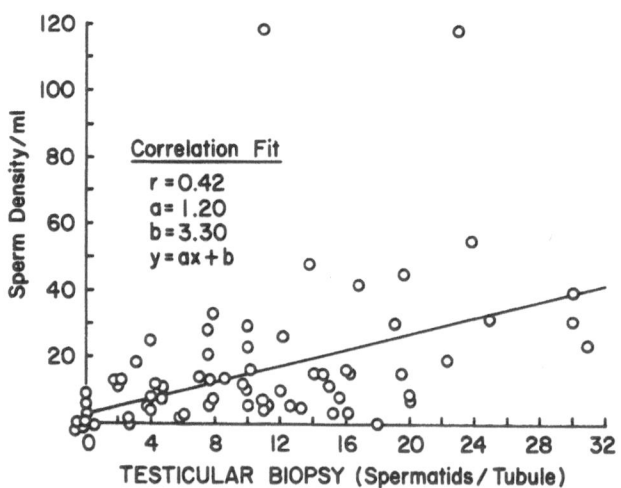

Figure 3   Correlation diagram of sperm density vs. spermatids per tubule on biopsy

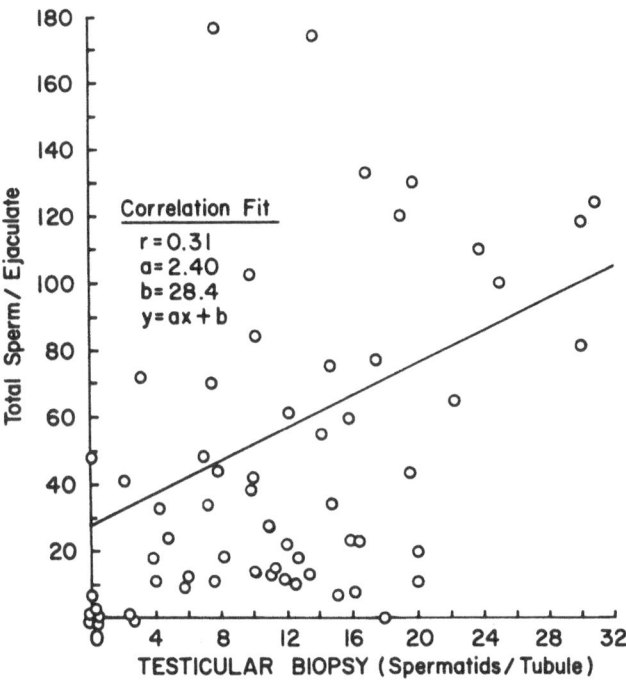

Figure 4 Correlation diagram of total sperm/ejaculate vs. spermatids/tubule on biopsy

Table 2 Spermatid counts in 39 men with 'normal' FSH and $> 10 \times 10^6$ sperm/ejaculate

Spermatids			
	<5/Tubule	-10	(25.6%)
	6–10/Tubule	- 7	(18.1%)
	11–15/Tubule	-10	(25.6%)
	> 16/Tubule	-12	(30.7%)
		39	(100.0%)

Mean 11.2 ± 7.9 Spermatids/Tubule

Table 3 Spermatid counts in 25 severely oligozoospermic men ($<10 \times 10^6$ sperm/ejaculate) with 'normal' FSH

Spermatids			
	0/tubule	- 8	(32%)
	1–5/Tubule	- 4	(16%)
	6–10/Tubule	- 4	(16%)
	> 11/Tubule	- 9	(36%)*
		25	(100%)

* 7 with documented ductal obstruction

83

DISCUSSION

Advances in the treatment of male infertility, such as microsurgery and gonadotropic stimulation, have made it imperative that every male with hypo-fertility be completely evaluated and given every chance for improved fertility. Just as it is no longer justified to 'write off' the severely oligozoo-spermic man, it behoves the urologist to pursue the aetiology, and properly classify hypofertility to the end that proper treatment may be selected.

Patients with severe oligozoospermia and elevated FSH may properly be referred for AIH (pending improvements in *in vitro* fertilization technology). However, in this age of cost-consciousness, serum FSH should be reserved for those with sperm counts below 15 million/ml or 50 million/ejaculate.

Genital duct obstruction should be considered in all azoospermic men with normal FSH and (from this series) in those with sperm counts up to 10 million/ejaculate (low semen volume, absent fructose, and lack of coagulation not withstanding). In such instances, *quantitative* testicular biopsy is essential. Silber[1] cites spermatid counts of 20 per tubule as 'normal' with an exponential correlation curve; however, in that series only 21 patients without ductal obstruction were evaluated. Assuming that 'normal' lies somewhere between 10 (present series) and 20 spermatids/tubule a standard can be established, nonetheless, below which, under strict circumstances, the epididymis should be examined for obstruction or the vas deferens evaluated radiologically.

In circumstances where serum FSH is normal in the face of oligozoospermia with severe hypospermatogenesis (Table 2) and no objective evidence of tubular obstruction (i.e. epididymal dilation), gonadotropin stimulation can rationally be attempted.

The difficulties (time involved, complexity) inherent in the objective analysis of testicular biopsy material are underscored in the comprehensive analysis of Pierrepoint *et al.*[2], and Zukerman *et al.*[3]. The method of Silber[1] is simple and is easily extended to the community hospital pathology department; however, even further objectivity is on the horizon in the form of DNA flow cytometry as described by Lipshultz[4].

References

1. Silber, S. J. and Rodriguez-Rigau, L. J. (1981). Quantitative analysis of testicle biopsy: Determination of partial obstruction and prediction of sperm count after surgery for obstruction. *Fertil. Steril.*, **36**, 480
2. Pierrepoint, C. G., Jenkins, B. N., Wilson, D. W., Phillips, M. J., Gow, J. G. (1982). An examination of blood steroid and gonadotropin concentrations in relation to fertility status and testicular function in men. *Fertil. Steril.*, **38**, 465
3. Zukerman, Z., Rodriguez, Rigau, L. J., Weis, D. B., Chowdhury, L. J., Smith, K. D. and Steinberger, E. (1978). Quantitative analysis of the seminiferous epithelium in human testicular biopsies, and the relation of spermatogenesis to sperm density. *Fertil. Steril.*, **30**, 448
4. Lipshultz, L. I. (1983). Update: New aspects in the diagnosis of male infertility. *Fertil. News*, **17**, 3

17
Response to FSH of human Sertoli cells in culture

V. SANTIEMMA, N. CASASANTA, P. ROSATI, S. MOSCARDELLI,
G. IAPADRE and A. FABBRINI

INTRODUCTION

The study of the Sertoli cell was greatly enhanced by the setting up in the mid 1970s of methods for the separation and culture of these cells. Since then many aspects of Sertoli cell function have been delineated. The Sertoli cell is a target for both FSH and androgens, has a steroid metabolizing activity and secretes testis specific proteins, such as ABP and inhibin[1], and also serum proteins[2].

However, all these pieces of information are relative to rat Sertoli cells, and little is known about human Sertoli cells. We report here an initial characterization of human Sertoli cell function in culture.

MATERIALS AND METHODS

Testes obtained from patients, aged 60–79 years who underwent surgical castration were finely minced, and the Sertoli cells were isolated according to the method of Steinberger[3], modified. The procedure consisted of a two-step enzymatic digestion first in 0.1% trypsin, and then in 0.25% collagenase at 37 °C. The incubation was carried out in a shaker bath at 150 shakes/min. After passing the supernatant through a wire mesh sieve (mesh size 120 μm) Sertoli cell clusters were primarily obtained. The cells were concentrated by centrifugation at 800 g for 5 min, resuspended in minimum essential medium (MEM) enriched with 4 mmol/l glutamine, 5% fetal calf serum, penicillin 100 IU/ml, streptomycin 100 μg/ml, plated in 60 mm petri-dishes, and incubated

85

at 34 °C under an atmosphere of 5% CO_2 and 25% O_2. In all experiments the medium was removed after 24 h and serum-free medium was used thereafter. Cultures consisted of approximately 80% Sertoli cells and 20% germ cells as determined by light microscopy.

At day 3 the medium was again changed, and a 30 min incubation was carried out to evaluate the cAMP response to FSH (10 μg/ml, NIH-FSH-B-1), MIX (1 mmol/l), LH (10 μg/ml, NIH-LH-S-18). At the end of incubation, cells were scraped and sonicated and the cAMP was evaluated by radio-immunoassay according to the method of Steiner et al. [4]. At day 4, other dishes (four per group) were incubated with the above mentioned hormones, plus testosterone (T, 0.5 μmol/l) alone or in combination, to determine the oestradiol production. The medium was removed after 24 h of incubation and stored at −20 °C. Oestradiol was evaluated by radioimmunoassay according to the method of De Alojsio et al. [5]. Proteins were measured by the method of Lowry [6].

RESULTS

Morphological aspect of human Sertoli cells in culture

Sertoli cells incubated in serum supplemented medium attached to the culture

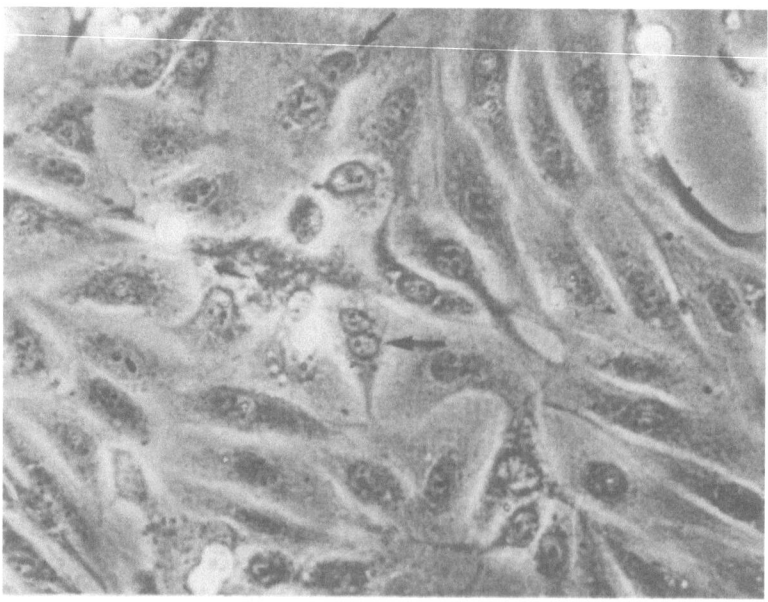

Figure 1 Monolayer of human Sertoli cells. Arrow heads indicate tripartite nucleoli. Phase contrast.   × 225

dish within 2–3 h of plating, and a confluent monolayer was identified by 24–36 h. The cells had a polygonal shape and their cytoplasm contained many vacuoles and granules (Figure 1), similar to those characteristic of rat Sertoli cells. The ovoid nucleus showed an evident nucleolus, often present in a tripartite complex (Figure 1) similar to that of rodent Sertoli cells.

Response to FSH

cAMP

MIX and LH did not induce any significant change in the cAMP concentration, nor did it with FSH alone. But FSH–MIX induced a significant cAMP response (Figure 2).

Oestradiol

Both T and FSH alone enhanced oestradiol secretion in comparison to the control but T was much more effective. However, the Sertoli cell aromatizing activity in the presence of the substrate was still increased by FSH (Figure 3).

DISCUSSION

Adult human Sertoli cells in culture respond to FSH with a rise in cAMP, confirming both that the cultured cell are Sertoli cells, and that human, like

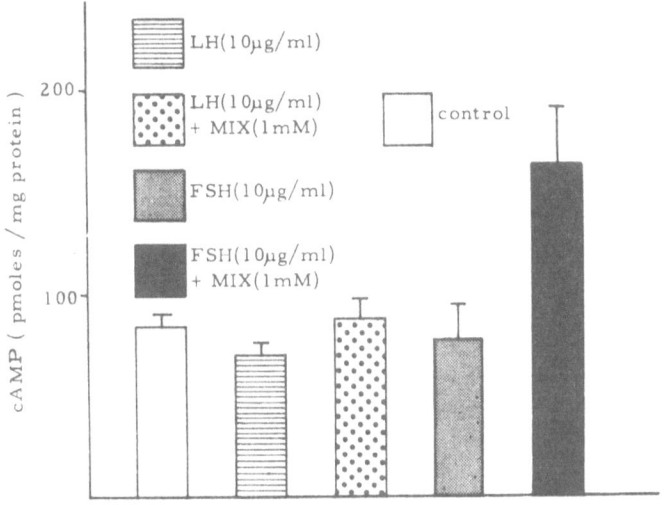

Figure 2 cAMP response in human Sertoli cells to FSH and LH stimulation

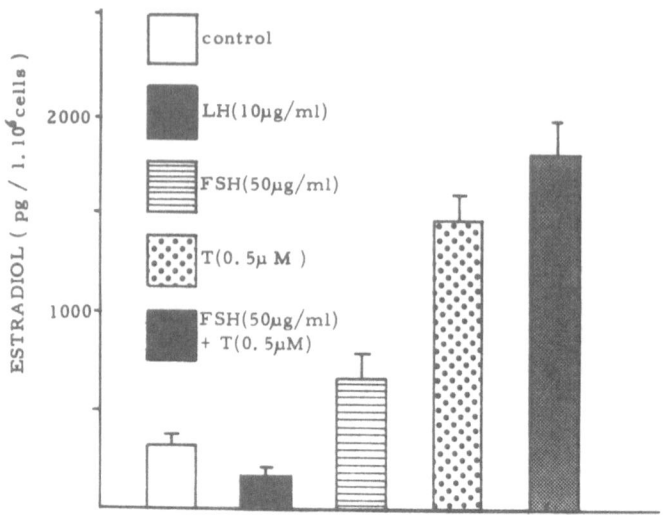

Figure 3 Oestradiol secretion in the presence of substrate and FSH

other mammalian, Sertoli cells are responsive to FSH. The order of magnitude of the response to FSH – about a two-fold increase in cAMP – is similar to that reported for the adult rat[7] and for human testicular biopsies[8], and definitely lower than that reported for the immature rat[7]. Thus the responsiveness of adult human Sertoli cells to FSH is blunted, and all the questions concerning the role of FSH in the adult rat and the mechanisms by which the response to FSH is turned off are open also to man. It has been reported that in the rat Sertoli cell responsiveness to FSH changes in the different stages of spermatogenesis, and is at its maximum at stages II–VI[9]. In man similar observations will be difficult to reproduce since spermatogenesis is not synchronized in waves, and no single tract of seminiferous tubules will show a single stage of spermatogenesis.

The intratesticular site of aromatization in man is a matter of controversy. Greater aromatase activity was found in whole testicular homogenates than in homogenates of seminiferous tubules, suggesting that this enzyme complex is present in interstitital tissue in man[10]. In addition, both Leydig and Sertoli cell tumours have been reported to secrete oestrogens[11]. Recently serum FSH and not LH was found to be a strong predictor of intratesticular oestradiol[12].

Our data on oestradiol secretion by cultured Sertoli cells suggest that the adult human Sertoli cell has an aromatizing activity, which is partially FSH-dependent. In the rat the FSH-dependent aromatase activity of the Sertoli cell has been reported only up to 3 weeks of age. Thus the proposed model of a local feed-back existing between Sertoli and Leydig cells, based on the negative influence of oestradiol on testosterone production, seems to be more suitable to man.

ACKNOWLEDGEMENT

We are greatly indebted to Dr F. Ledda of the Urological Clinic, University of Chieti, for providing the orchidectomy material.

References

1. Ritzén, E. M., Hansson, V. and French, F. S. (1981). The Sertoli cell. In Burger, H. and Dekretser, D. (eds.) *The Testis.* pp. 171–194 (New York: Raven Press)
2. Wright, W. W., Musto, N. A., Mather, P. and Bardin, C. W. (1981). Sertoli cells secrete both testis specific and serum proteins. *Proc. Natl. Acad. Sci., USA,* **78,** 7565
3. Steinberger, A., Lindsey, N., Heindel, J. J., Sanborn, B. and Elkington, S. H. (1975). Isolation and culture of FSH-responsive Sertoli cells. *Endocrinol. Res. Commun.,* **2,** 261
4. Steiner, A. L., Parker, C. W. and Kipnis, D. M. (1972). Radioimmunoassay for cyclic nucleotides. *J. Biol. Chem.,* **247,** 1100
5. De Alojsio, D., Fraticelli, A., Bolelli, G. F., Vecchi, F. and Bianchini, C. (1975). Basal values and circadian variations of testosterone, estradiol, FSH and LH in the plasma of normal adult males. *Acta Eur. Fertil.,* **6,** 52
6. Lowry, O. H., Rosebrough, N. J., Furr, A. L. and Randall, R. J. (1951). Protein measurement with the folin phenol reagent. *J. Biol. Chem.,* **193,** 265
7. Steinberger, A., Mintz, M. and Heindel, J. J. (1978). Changes in cyclic AMP response to FSH in isolated rat Sertoli cells during sexual maturation. *Biol. Reprod.,* **19,** 566
8. Heindel, J. J., Lipshultz, L. I. and Steinberger, E. (1978). Stimulation of cyclic AMP accumulation in human testes *in vitro* by LH, FSH and prostaglandins. *Fertil. Steril.,* **30,** 595
9. Parvinen, M., Marana, R., Robertson, D. M., Hansson, V. and Ritzen, E. M. (1980). Functional cycle of rat Sertoli cells: differential binding and action of FSH at various stages of the spermatogenetic cycle. In Steinberger, A. and Steinberger, E. (eds.) *Testicular Development, Structure and Function.* pp. 425–32. (New York: Raven Press)
10. Payne, A. H., Kelch, R. P., Musich, S. S. and Holpern, M. E. (1976). Intratesticular site of aromatization in the human. *J. Clin. Endocrinol. Metab.,* **42,** 1081
11. De Jong, F. H., Hey, A. H. and Van der Molen, H. J. (1974). Estradiol-17β and testosterone in rat testis tissue: effect of gonadotropins, localization and production *in vitro. J. Endocrinol.,* **60,** 409
12. Takahashi, J., Higashu, Y., Lanasa, J. A., Winters, S. J., Oshima, H. and Troen, P. (1982). Studies of the human testis. XVII. Gonadotropin regulation of intratesticular testosterone and estradiol in infertile men. *J. Clin. Endocrinol. Metab.,* **55,** 1073

18
Anaerobic urinary and prostatic bacteria, and prostatic biochemical markers in urine after prostatic massage of infertile men

P. J. MOBERG, P. ENEROTH, J. LIZANA and C. E. NORD

INTRODUCTION

The importance of a chronic genital tract infection has been recognized as a possible cause of male infertility[1]. The diagnosis of a chronic male genital tract infection is based, apart from semen analyses, on palpatory findings of the prostatic gland, the occurrence of an increased number of leukocytes in EPS (expressed prostatic secretion) or in a urinary sediment obtained after prostatic massage, and finally on bacteriological analyses of ejaculates[2]. There is, however, a considerable lack of agreement between these different methods used for diagnosing a male adnexitis[3,4]. It has been reported that saline dilution of semen has resulted in increased bacterial growth by decreasing the inhibitory effect on bacteria exerted by prostatic secretions[2]. Whether urine can exert a similar inhibitory effect is not known.

The aim of the present investigation was to study the occurrence of anaerobic and aerobic bacteria in urine voided before and after prostatic massage of infertile men. The results of such a study might be of greater importance if the admixture of EPS to urine voided after prostatic massage could be assessed by simultaneous analyses of prostatic biochemical markers[5], i.e. prostatic acid phosphatase (PAP), β_2-microglobulin (β_2-m), carcinoembryonic antigen (CEA) and albumin.

MATERIALS AND METHODS

Twenty-five men (age 21–42 years) whose wives had consulted the Department of Obstetrics and Gynaecology were included in the study. Seven of the men had a previous paternity and 11 had been previously treated for a urogenital tract infection. None of the men had received antibiotics during the preceding 3 months. The men delivered a urine sample before (U1) and after (U2) massage of the prostate. EPS was obtained from 11 men. Samples of urine and EPS were immediately cultured on blood agar plates aerobically and anaerobically, and urine was also injected into an anaerobic gas transport bottle. The culture and identification of bacteria was carried out as described elsewhere[6]. The remaining urine was frozen and stored until analysed by radioimmunoassay (RIA; β_2-m (kit from Pharmacia, Sweden); CEA (CIS, France); PAP (NEN, USA)). Albumin was determined by immuno-nephelometry[7].

RESULTS

There was a significant increase in the number of anaerobic bacterial isolates in urine voided after prostatic massage (Table 1). The bacterial species most frequently isolated in samples of U1 and U2 are seen in Table 2. 95% of the isolates tested for susceptibility to doxycycline were sensitive in concentrations which can be expected to be found in prostatic secretion.

There was an increase in PAP concentration in U2 as compared to U1 in all patients (Table 3). If PAP in urine represents a true marker of prostatic secretion then β_2-m seems to be a useful prostatic marker.

Table 1 Number of aerobic and anaerobic bacterial isolates in urine voided before and after massage of the prostate

| | Number of bacterial isolates | | |
	Aerobic	Anaeobic	Total
Urine voided *before* prostatic massage	12	21	33
Urine voided *after* prostatic massage	16	43	59

Table 2 Most frequent anaerobic bacterial species in urine voided before and after prostatic massage

Bacterial species	Before prostatic massage Number of patients	After prostatic massage Number of patients
Peptostreptococcus micros	1	4
Peptococcus asacharolyticus	2	6
Eubacterium lentum	3	9
Bacteroides species	1	6

Table 3 Mean compound concentrations and relative number of patients with increased compound concentrations in urine voided after massage of the prostate

Compound analysed		U1	U2	Frequencies of increased compound concentrations	%
PAP	$\mu g/l$	5	46	25/25	100
β_2-m	$\mu g/l$	168	378	24/25	96
CEA	$\mu g/1$	12	22	17/25	68
Albumin	mg/l	14	22	21/25	84

CONCLUSION

Two types of finding could be observed.

(1) Evident increase of prostatic acid phosphatase (PAP) and β_2-m in urine voided after prostatic massage combined with an absence of increase in the number of bacterial species.

(2) Evident increase of PAP and β_2-m in urine voided after prostatic massage combined with the presence of an increased number of bacterial species.

The findings of type (1) probably show that there is no infection, whereas findings of type (2) indicate a bacterial infection in the prostate and/or surrounding tissues. The combination of bacterial and prostatic biochemical marker analyses may be useful in the clinical evaluation of male infertility.

References

1. McGowan, M. P., Burger, H. G., Baker, H. W. G., de Kretser, D. M. and Kovacs, G. (1981). The incidence of non-specific infection in the semen in fertile and subfertile males. Int. J. Androl., 4, 657
2. Comhaire, F., Verschraegen, G. and Vermeulen, L. (1980). Diagnosis of accessory gland infection and its possible role in male infertility. Int. J. Androl., 3, 32
3. Johanisson, E. and Eliasson, R. (1978). Cytological studies of prostatic fluid from men with and without abnormal palpatory findings of the prostate. Int. J. Androl., 1, 201
4. Colpi, G. M., Zanollo, A., Roveda, M. L., Tomasini-Degna, A. and Baretta, G. (1982). Anaerobic and aerobic bacteria in secretions of the prostate and seminal vesicles of infertile men. Arch. Androl., 9, 175
5. Lizana, J., Moberg, P. J. and Eneroth, P. (1983). Beta$_2$-microglobulin, carcinoembryonic antigen and prostate acid phosphatase in split ejaculates and urine voided before and after massage of the prostate. Arch. Androl., 11, 225
6. Moberg, P. J., Gottlieb, C. and Nord, C. G. (1982). Anaerobic bacteria in uterine infection following first trimester abortion. Eur. J. Clin. Microbiol., 1, 82
7. Lizana, J. and Blad, E. (1983). Immunonephelometry of specific proteins in human seminal plasma. Clin. Chem., 29, 618

19
Effects of bombesin on the pituitary response to TRH and LHRH in humans

C. SCARPIGNATO, G. BAIO and A. E. PONTIROLI

INTRODUCTION

Bombesin, a tetradecapeptide originally isolated from amphibian skin, is now considered as a putative mammalian neuropeptide[1]. Indeed, bombesin-like immunoreactivity is distributed throughout the brain, with the highest concentration in the hypothalamus[2,3]. These bombesin-like components are localized to synaptosomes and are released from hypothalamic slices by depolarizing stimuli in a Ca^{2+}-dependent manner[4]. The presence of bombesin-like peptides in the hypothalamus, and their secretion from hypothalamic nerve endings, suggest that they may be released into the portal blood and may affect pituitary function. As a matter of fact, some authors (for review see ref. 5) found that intravenous or intracerebral administration of bombesin and/or GRP* modifies the secretion of some anterior pituitary hormones. Results of the present investigation suggest that this neuropeptide may have a role in the control of *human* pituitary secretion.

MATERIALS AND METHODS

Six male healthy volunteers (average age 24 years) participated in the study after written informed consent. The tests were performed after an overnight fast and abstinence from smoking. At about 0900 h two 19 gauge butterflies were

---

* Gastrin Releasing Peptide, a heptacosapeptide isolated from porcine non-antral tissue which presents in its C-terminal decapeptide structural similarities with the amphibian bombesin.

inserted into the antecubital veins: one for the administration of the peptide, the other for blood sampling. Patency was preserved by a slow infusion of physiological saline. After withdrawal of three basal blood samples (-90, -75 and -60 min), bombesin† (5 ng kg^{-1} min^{-1}) or saline was infused on 2 different days and in random order. The infusion began at -60 min and continued for 150 min. At zero time the hypothalamic releasing hormones (200 μg of TRH and 100 μg of LHRH) were injected together as a bolus. Afterwards, additional blood samples were drawn. Plasma prolactin, TSH, LH and FSH were assayed with specific RIAs as previously described[6], by using Biodata reagents. Quantitative evaluation of hormone production was made by calculating the area under the curves of immunoreactivity in plasma after subtraction of basal values. All values were presented as a mean ± SE. Student's t-test was used to determine statistical significance between secretory areas.

RESULTS

Results obtained in the present investigation are summarized in Figure 1 which depicts the integrated response of the four hormones studied. Though bombesin had no effect on basal levels of prolactin, TSH, LH and FSH, it modified the pituitary response to TRH and LHRH.

DISCUSSION

Results of the present investigation demonstrate that intravenous administration of bombesin modifies the pituitary response to exogenously administered releasing factors, without affecting the basal values of all the hormones studied.

The site at which bombesin acts to alter pituitary hormone release is unknown. Previous studies[5] have indicated that the endocrine effects of various peptides can be exerted by an action on the hypothalamus and/or on the pituitary. As far as bombesin is concerned, it was demonstrated that, when incubated with rat hemipituitaries *in vitro*, this peptide is able to stimulate LH and FSH release[7]. In addition, bombesin was able to stimulate prolactin and GH release in human pituitary tumour cultures[8]. These data and the high concentration of bombesin-like immunoreactivity present in the hypothalamus strongly suggest a direct effect of the peptide at pituitary level.

The mechanism by which bombesin modifies the secretion of pituitary hormones is also unknown. Some effects of bombesin, like those on gastric secretion[9] and on gastric motility[10], appear to be antagonized by opioids: thus an interaction between bombesin and endogenous opioid peptides (EOP) may be hypothesized. Indeed, bombesin induces the same modifications as

† Gift from Dr Chiara De Paolis (Farmitalia-Carlo Erba Research Laboratories, Milan, Italy)

naloxone in the pituitary secretions studied[11]. Because evidence has been presented indicating that levels of EOP in the hypothalamus may help to regulate normal pituitary hormone secretion[11], an action of bombesin on the hypophysis through an antagonism towards EOP might be postulated.

Previous data and results of the present investigation support the idea that both types of peptides (bombesin-like peptides and EOP), present in high concentrations in the hypothalamus, may be involved in the physiological control of pituitary hormone secretion.

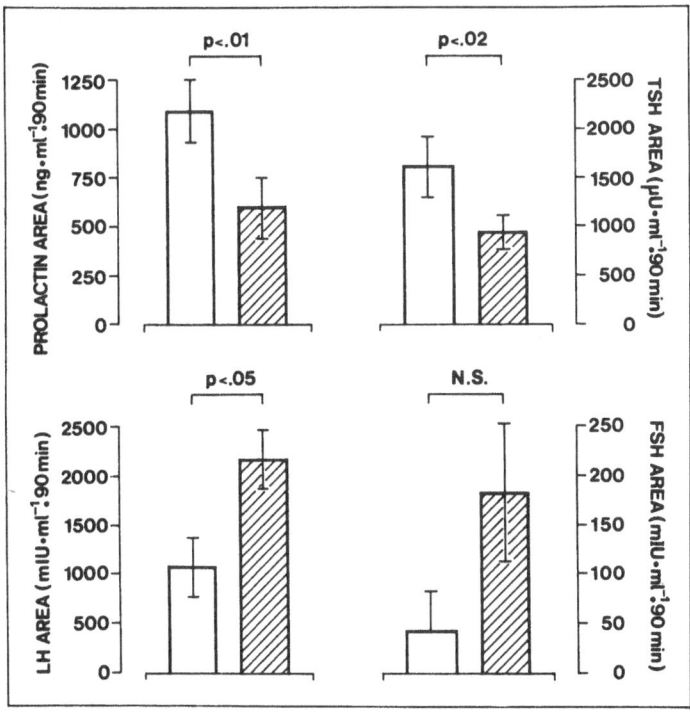

Figure 1 Secretory areas of prolactin, TSH, LH and TRH during saline (white columns) or bombesin (hatched columns) infusion. Each column represents the mean of the values obtained from six subjects. Vertical bars are standard errors.

ACKNOWLEDGEMENT

This work was supported by grants from CNR and MPI (Rome).

References

1. Brown, M. and Vale, W. (1979). Bombesin – a putative mammalian neurogastrointestinal peptide. *Trends Neuro. Sci.*, **2**, 95

2. Brown, M., Allen, R., Villareal, J. and Vale, W. (1978). Bombesin-like activity: radio-immunologic assessment in biologic tissues. *Life Sci.*, **23**, 2721
3. Moody, T. W., Thoa, N. B., O'Donohue, T. L. and Pert, C. B. (1980). Bombesin-like peptides in rat brain: quantitation and biochemical characterization. *Biochem. Biophys. Res. Comm.*, **90**, 7
4. Moody, T. W., Thoa, N. N., O'Donohue, T. L. and Pert, C. B. (1980). Bombesin-like peptides: localization in synaptosomes and release from hypothalamic tissues. *Life Sci.*, **26**, 1707
5. McCann, S. M. (1980). Control of anterior pituitary hormone release by brain peptides. *Neuroendocrinology*, **31**, 335
6. Pontiroli, A. E., Alberetto, M., Restelli, L. and Facchinetti, A. (1980). Effect of bombesin and ceruletide on prolactin, growth hormone, luteinizing hormone and parathyroid hormone release in normal human males. *J. Clin. Endocrinol. Metab.*, **51**, 1303
7. Morley, J. E., Briggs, J. E., Solomon, T. E., Melmed, S., Lamers, C., Damassa, D. A., Carlson, H. E. and Hershman, J. M. (1979). Cholecystokinin-octapeptide releases growth hormone from rat pituitaries *in vitro*. *Life Sci.*, **25**, 1201.
8. White, M. C., Adams, E. A. and Mashiter, K. (1981). Effect of CCK and bombesin on PRL and GH secretion in human pituitary tumour cultures. *Acta Endocrinol.*, **97** (Suppl. 243), 251
9. Materia, A., Jaffe, B. M., Modlin, I. M., Sank, A. and Albert, D. (1982). Effect of methionine-enkephalin and naloxone on bombesin-stimulated gastric acid secretion, gastrin and pancreatic polypeptide release in the dog. *Ann. Surg.*, **196**, 48
10. Zetler, G. (1980). Antagonism of the gut-contracting effect of bombesin and neurotensin by opioid peptides, morphine, atropine or tetrodotoxin. *Pharmacology*, **21**, 348
11. Meites, J., Bruni, J. F., Van Vugt, D. A. and Smith, A. (1979). Relation of endogenous opioid peptides and morphine to neuroendocrine functions. *Life Sci.*, **24**, 1325

Section 3

Immunology and
Male Reproduction

20
Characteristics of a monoclonal anti-human sperm antibody

V. BAUKLOH, S. PAUL and L. METTLER

INTRODUCTION

With the aim of elucidating the applicability of anti-human sperm antibodies as fertility regulators[1] monoclonal antibodies were generated and tested for their individual potentials. From 149 hybridoma cell lines secreting anti-sperm antibodies one – hereafter referred to as III 3 – was studied in detail.

MATERIALS AND METHODS

The generation of monoclonal antibodies against PBS washed intact human spermatozoa was carried out as previously described[2]. Supernatants of cell colonies developing from fused splenocytes × myeloma cells, as well as human sera containing naturally occurring sperm antibodies were tested for antibody production or concentration by an enzyme linked immunosorbent assay (ELISA)[3] against immobilized sperm and seminal plasma. For specificity tests and evaluation of antigenic potencies the ELISA was modifed by addition of a competing antigen to the fluid tested against intact sperm.

High titre antibodies from selected cell lines were obtained as ascites fluids by injection of cells into pristane primed Balb/c mice.

Sera from infertility patients were provided by the WHO reference bank in Aarhus, Denmark. Those applied in competitive ELISA exhibited reactivity with human spermatozoa in ELISA and in the tray agglutination[4] and immobilization[5] assays. Ascites fluid of monoclonal antibody III 3 was also subjected to the tray agglutination and immobilization tests.

The corresponding antigen of the studied antibody was purified from seminal plasma according to the method reported earlier[6] by immunoaffinity chromatography. Eluted fractions were tested for their ability to inhibit the reactivity of III 3 antibody with immobilized sperm in competitive ELISA. The purity of the isolated antigen was checked by polyacrylamide gel (PAG) electrophoresis. Localization of the antigen reactive with III 3 antibody on the sperm surface and on test tissues was carried out by the immunoperoxidase technique.

RESULTS

The monoclonal antibody III 3, in the form of mouse ascites fluid, exhibited marked agglutinating and immobilizing activity against living human spermatozoa. Therefore, sperm specificity was suspected and the isolation of the corresponding antigen initiated. Immunoaffinity chromatography revealed two peaks (Figure 1) which inhibited the ELISA reactivity of III 3 antibody with immobilized sperm. PAG electrophoresis of the eluted peaks showed a single protein band indicating one homogeneous antigen. The antigenic potency of the purified antigen, with regard to the inhibition of III 3 antibody reaction with intact sperm, was 65.1 fold that of seminal plasma.

In a competitive ELISA the reactivity of the antigen III 3 with naturally

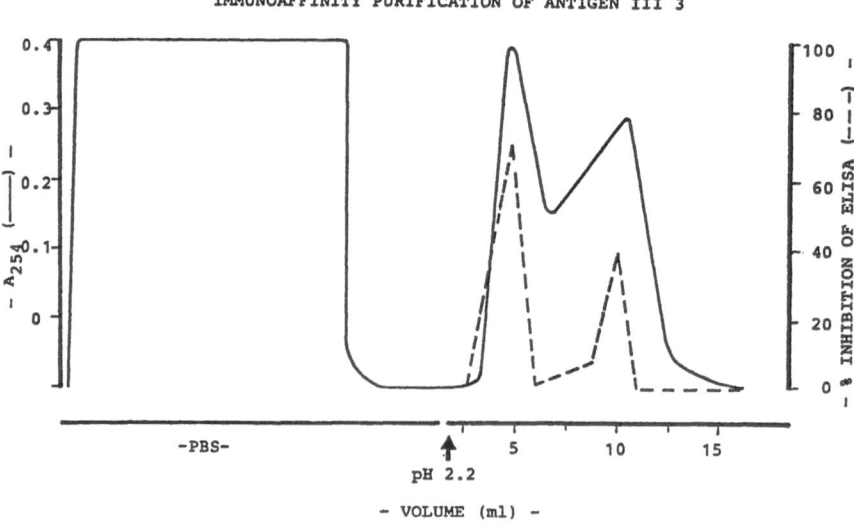

Figure 1   Isolation of the antigen reactive with the antibody III 3. Elution was performed with glycine-HCl buffer, pH 2.2, and the fractions obtained were tested for their ability to inhibit the reactivity of III 3 antibody with immobilized sperm in competitive ELISA

Table 1   Reactivity of the III 3 antigen with naturally occurring anti-human sperm antibodies

	0–25	25–50	% Inhibition* 50–75	75–100
No. of sera (n=34)	7	11	10	6

* Sera were assayed for sperm reactivity in ELISA with (10 μg) and without purified III 3 antigen. Results were computed after correction for non-specific binding.

occurring anti-sperm antibodies in sera of infertility patients was tested (Table 1). Seven out of 34 sera were found to be weakly to non-reactive while the sperm reactivity of 16 was strongly inhibited (> 50%) by the presence of III 3 antigen. Detailed cross-reactivity tests with the antibody III 3 against a panel of human tissues revealed the presence of the III 3 antigen on placental endothelium and on a subpopulation of peripheral T-lymphocytes. In order to test if antigen shedding of III 3 does occur, the concentration of the free antigen in seminal plasma and in human sera was examined. Levels in seminal plasma ranged from 282–475 μg III 3 antigen per ml, in sera concentration of 13.4–18.1 μg were detected.

DISCUSSION

The high agglutinating and immobilizing activity of the investigated monoclonal anti-human antibody III 3, and the high percentage of sera from infertility patients (79% in total) reacting with the corresponding purified antigen to at least 25% indicate that the sperm surface antigen III 3 plays a role in the induction of natural antibody production against spermatozoa. Nevertheless, this antigen is not sperm specific as demonstrated by the immunoperoxidase staining of a subpopulation of T-lymphocytes after incubation with III 3 antibody. The III 3 antigen appears to be loosely bound to, and easily shed from, the surfaces of spermatozoa and T-lymphocytes, since considerable concentrations of the free antigen were detected in both seminal plasma and serum.

In conclusion, the spermatozoal antigen III 3, probably important for antibody production initiation *in vivo*, is not a candiate for immunological fertility control. Further studies to identify biologically active and sperm specific monoclonal antibodies are, therefore, under way.

References

1. Goldberg, E. (1979). Sperm specific antigens and immunological approaches for control of fertility. In *Recent Advances in Reproduction and Regulation of Fertility*, p. 281. (Elsevier: North Holland Biomedical Press)
2. Paul, S., Baukloh, V., Baillie, M. and Mettler, L. (1982). Generation of monoclonal antibodies against human spermatozoa and seminal plasma constituents. *Clin. Reprod. Fertil.*, 1, 235
3. Paul, S., Baukloh, V. and Mettler, L. (1983). Enzyme-linked immunosorbent assays for sperm antibody detection and antigenic analysis. *J. Immunol. Meth.*, 56, 193
4. Friberg, J. (1974). Immunological studies on sperm-agglutinating sera from women. *Acta Obstet. Gynecol. Scand.*, 36, 21
5. Hustedt, T. and Hjort, T. (1974). Microtechnique for detection of sperm-immobilization and cytotoxity. *WHO-Workshop of Iso- and Auto-Antibodies to Human Spermatozoa.* 15–19 July, Aarhus
6. Paul, S., Baukloh, V., Czuppon, A. B. and Mettler, L. (1983). The use of monoclonal antibodies against human spermatozoa for the isolation and identification of sperm-specific antigens. In *Immunological Factors in Human Contraception*, p. 103. Field Educational Italia Acta Medica

21
Topographical analysis of the surface of human spermatozoa by means of monoclonal antibodies

A. C. HINRICHSEN, M. J. HINRICHSEN and W.-B. SCHILL

INTRODUCTION

Mammalian spermatozoa emerge highly differentiated from the testis, but continue to develop during their passage through the epididymis, acquiring a mature motility pattern and fertilizing ability[1-4]. This process, termed sperm maturation, involves a series of morphological and biochemical modifications which are particularly obvious in the sperm membrane system[5]. A review of the subject indicates that agents produced and secreted by the epithelial cells lining the epididymal duct are the most likely to be involved in this process[6-10].

The spermatozoan membrane system is also implicated in other important transformations which this cell undergoes following ejaculation in the female reproductive tract. Thus, spermatozoa undergo a process termed capacitation, whereby the sperm cell surface components suffer a series of modifications such as loss and/or reorganization of the surface glycoproteins[9,11,12]. This process leads then to the occurrence of the acrosome reaction which takes place just before or during the passage of the spermatozoa through the investments of the oocyte[13].

Which factors on the spermatozoan membrane system play an important role during these events, and which are responsible for the resulting sperm-egg attachment and interaction during fertilization are still unknown. The complexity of the spermatozoan membrane system[14] has rendered the elucidation of its structure and function difficult by means of the conventional biochemical and immunological methods[15,16]. This has led us to adopt the method of monoclonal antibody production[17] for the characterization and identification of those factors involved in the different events leading to fertilization[18].

MATERIALS AND METHODS

Human spermatozoa were obtained from patients attending our Andrology Unit. Only those ejaculates presenting a normal morphology ($<30\%$ pathological forms), 60–70% motile spermatozoa, and more than 50×10^6 cells/ml were considered adequate for our purposes. The ejaculates were diluted 1:1 in HEPES buffer, pH 7.2, carefully layered on 7.5% Ficoll, and centrifuged. Under these conditions, spermatozoa were freed of all residues of seminal plasma and remained morphologically and functionally intact, as was determined by their ability to penetrate zona pellucida-free hamster oocytes. The pelleted spermatozoa were pooled and the resulting suspension was injected intraperitoneally and subcutaneously in female Balb/c mice in Freund's complete adjuvant. The animals were boostered after 10 days and further immunized every 2 weeks over a period of 16–20 weeks in order to obtain predominantly IgG and not IgM producing clones. Immunological response was periodically checked in the serum of the immunized mice by means of an enzyme-linked immunoassay (ELISA). Briefly, whole washed spermatozoa were bound on poly-L-lysine coated microtitre plates and incubated with the serum to be tested, followed by an incubation with an anti-mouse Ig antibody labelled with alkaline phosphatase.

The spleen cells from mice producing anti-sperm antibodies were then fused with NS-1 mouse myeloma cells in the presence of polyethylene glycol, and the resulting hybridoma cell suspension was cloned in HAT-selection medium. Anti-sperm antibody production was screened 10 days after the fusion by means of the ELISA test. Anti-sperm antibody producing cultures were then subcloned in complete growth medium and further cultured.

RESULTS AND DISCUSSION

A total of 1457 different hybridoma cell lines were achieved following seven fusions, out of which 748 (51%) developed further over a period of 2–3 months following the corresponding fusion. Screening of the supernatants of these hybridoma cultures revealed that a total of 269 clones (18% of the original cultures) produced and secreted antibody against whole washed spermatozoa. Anti-sperm antibody producing clones were further characterized by means of indirect immunofluorescence. Table 1 summarizes the results obtained for the nine most interesting clones. Furthermore, we also determined, by means of

Table 1 Antibody subclass determination and indirect immunofluorescent analysis on washed human spermatozoa of the supernatants of nine hybridoma cell lines

Clone number	Ig-subclass	Immunofluorescence on washed human spermatozoa
G_{225}	IgG_{2a}	Acrosome
D_{81}	IgG_{2b}	Acrosome
D_3	IgG_1	Equatorial segment
F_4	IgG_{2a}	Equatorial segment + middle piece
G_{218}	IgG_{2b}	Acrosome
G_{112}	IgG_{2b}	Acrosome
G_{177}	IgG_{2a}	Acrosome + middle piece
G_{178}	IgG_1	Acrosome
G_{220}	IgG_{2b}	Acrosome + equatorial segment

the ELISA test, the subclass of the immunoglobulins secreted by these clones. A great part of the monoclonal antibodies produced by these clones recognized antigens on the acrosomal cap of human washed spermatozoa. Clones G_{177} and G_{220} secreted antibodies which additionally recognized antigens in the middle piece and in the equatorial segment, respectively. Immunofluorescence of the supernatants of clones D_3 and F_4 showed mainly reaction in the equatorial segment; in the case of clone F_4, a very faint reaction was also observed in the middle piece.

A further step in the characterization of our monoclonal antisperm antibodies was to determine their specificity for spermatozoa. For this purpose we tested the supernatants of our nine clones against seminal plasma by means of the ELISA test, in which case we coated the microtitre plates with seminal plasma, and against cryostat thin tissue sections of human liver, uterus, spleen, and ovary, by means of indirect immunofluorescence. Table 2

Table 2 Determination of the reactivity of the supernatants of nine hybridoma cell lines against washed human spermatozoa, seminal plasma, thin secretions of various tissues, and isolated acrosin

Clone number	Human spermatozoa	Seminal plasma	Other tissues	Isolated acrosin
G_{225}	+	−	−	+
D_{81}	+	−	−	+
D_3	+	−	−	−
F_4	+	−	−	−
G_{218}	+	−	−	+
G_{112}	+	−	−	+
G_{177}	+	−	−	±
G_{178}	+	−	−	+
G_{220}	+	−	−	−

summarizes the data obtained: no cross-reaction, whether with seminal plasma, nor with the thin sections of the tissues tested was observed, a result which stresses the specificity for spermatozoa of our anti-sperm antibodies. Furthermore, when tested by means of ELISA against isolated acrosin, five of these supernatants gave a strong positive reaction, one gave a faint positive reaction, and three were negative. It is worth pointing out that those acrosin-positive supernatants gave an intense fluorescence on the acrosomal cap.

It is our purpose to use these anti-human spermatozoa monoclonal antibodies as a tool for the characterization of the structure of the complex spermatozoan membrane system, and in particular to elucidate the biochemistry and physiology of its components. We hope thus to be able to better understand the molecular mechanism involved in the processes of epididymal sperm maturation, capacitation and fertilization. Furthermore, the high specificity of these antibodies will in the future probably allow their application as an effective and specific immunological contraceptive method.

ACKNOWLEDGEMENT

The authors appreciate the skilful technical assistance of Miss A. Weiss. This work was supported by a research grant from the Deutsche Forschungsgemeinschaft (Schi-86/7-3). A. C. Hinrichsen is a recipient of an Alexander von Humboldt Research Fellowship.

References

1. Young, W. C. (1931). A study of the function of the epididymis. III. Functional changes undergone by the spermatozoa during their passage through the epididymis and the vas deferens in the guinea pig. *J. Exp. Biol.*, **8**, 151
2. Blandau, R. J. and Rumery, R. E. (1964). The relationship of swimming movements of epididymal spermatozoa to their fertilizing ability. *Fertil. Steril.*, **15**, 571
3. Bedford, J. M. (1966). Development of the fertilizing ability of spermatozoa in the epididymis of the rabbit. *J. Exp. Biol.*, **163**, 319
4. Orgebin-Crist, M. C. (1967). Maturation of spermatozoa in the rabbit epididymis: fertilizing ability and embryonic mortality in does inseminated with epididymal spermatozoa. *Ann. Biol. Anim. Biochem. Biophys.*, **7**, 373
5. Hinrichsen-Kohane, A. C., Hinrichsen, M. J. and Schill, W.-B. (1984). Molecular events leading to fertilization – a review. *Andrologia*, 321
6. Lea, O. A., Petrusz, P. and French, F. S. (1978). Purification and localization of acidic epididymal glycoprotein (AEG): a sperm coating protein secreted by the rat epididymis. *Int. J. Androl.*, Suppl. 2, 592
7. Kohane, A. C., Garberi, J. C., Cameo, M. S. and Blaquier, J. A. (1979). Quantitative determination of specific proteins in the rat epididymis. *J. Steroid Biochem.*, **11**, 671
8. Kohane, A. C., Pineiro, L., Cameo, M. S., Garberi, J. C. and Blaquier, J. A. (1980). Distribution and site of production of specific proteins in the rat epididymis. *Biol. Reprod.*, **23**, 181
9. Kohane, A. C., Gonzalez-Echeverria, F. M. C., Pineiro, L. and Blaquier, J. A. (1980). The interaction of proteins of epididymal origin with spermatozoa. *Biol. Reprod.*, **23**, 737

10. Kohane, A. C., Pineiro, L. and Blaquier, J. A. (1983). Hormonal control of the synthesis of specific proteins in the rat epididymis. *Endocrinology*, **112**, 1590
11. Bedford, J. M. (1970). Sperm capacitation and fertilization in mammals. *Biol. Reprod.*, Suppl. 2, 128
12. Brackett, B. G. and Oliphant, G. (1975). Capacitation of rabbit spermatozoa *in vitro. Biol. Reprod.*, **12**, 260
13. Gwatkin, R. B. L. (1977). The acrosome reaction. In R. B. L. Gwatkin (ed.) *Fertilization Mechanisms in Man and Mammals*, p. 61. (New York: Plenum Press)
14. Töpfer-Petersen, E., Hinrichsen-Kohane, A. C. and Schill, W.-B. (1982). Immunological analysis of the boar spermatozoan outer acrosomal membrane. *Arch. Dermat. Res.*, **273**, 176
15. Töpfer-Petersen, E., Hinrichsen-Kohane, A. C., Schmoekel, C. and Schill, W.-B. (1984). The acrosomal membrane system and its role in mammalian fertilization. In W. Voelter, E. Bayer, Y. A. Orchinnikov, E. Wünsch (eds.) *Chemistry of Peptides and Proteins.* p. 363, vol. 2. (Berlin-New York: Walter de Gruyter)
16. Hinrichsen, A. C., Töpfer-Petersen, E. and Schill, W.-B. (1983). Immunological characterization of the outer acrosomal membrane of boar spermatozoa. (In preparation)
17. Köhler, G. and Milstein, C. (1975). Continuous cultures of fused cells secreting antibody of predefined specificity. *Nature*, **256**, 495
18. Hinrichsen, A. C., Hinrichsen, M. J. and Schill, W.-B. (1984). Analysis of antigen expression on human spermatozoa by means of monoclonal antibodies. *Fertil. Steril.* (In press)

22
Human seminal plasma proteins: identification and preliminary characterization of a human sperm coating antigen (h-SCA) protein in physiological and pathological conditions

G. LOMBARDI, M. DE ROSA, L. QUAGLIOZZI, M. MINOZZI [†],
P. ABRESCIA, J. GUARDIOLA and S. METAFORA

ABSTRACT

The presence in the human seminal plasma (h-SP) of a protein immunologically related to the RSV-IV, protein secreted by the rat seminal vesicles (RSV), is shown. We also report that this protein (hereafter termed the h-SCA protein) binds the human sperm cell surface. This protein has been partially characterized by chromatography and gel electrophoresis, and could represent a good marker to study the human function of seminal vesicles and their androgen regulation.

Due to the availability of a sensitive immunological assay for h-SCA, we were also able to analyse its expression in normal and pathological conditions. The results of the analysis suggest that low levels of testosterone are not associated with low levels of the h-SCA. On the other hand, since other pathological conditions, such as Klinefelter's syndrome, affect h-SCA levels more dramatically than testosterone concentrations it should be concluded that the expression of the h-SCA protein is regulated by multiple mechanisms, one of which could be testosterone dependent.

111

INTRODUCTION

The sperm-free, non-dialysable fraction of human semen has a complex composition and enzymology[1], and shows genetic polymorphisms[2]. These characteristics have been exploited for clinical studies of age-related changes, correlations between diseases and infertility, diagnosis of disease, and the physiology of reproduction, as well as in forensic science[3]. In this paper we

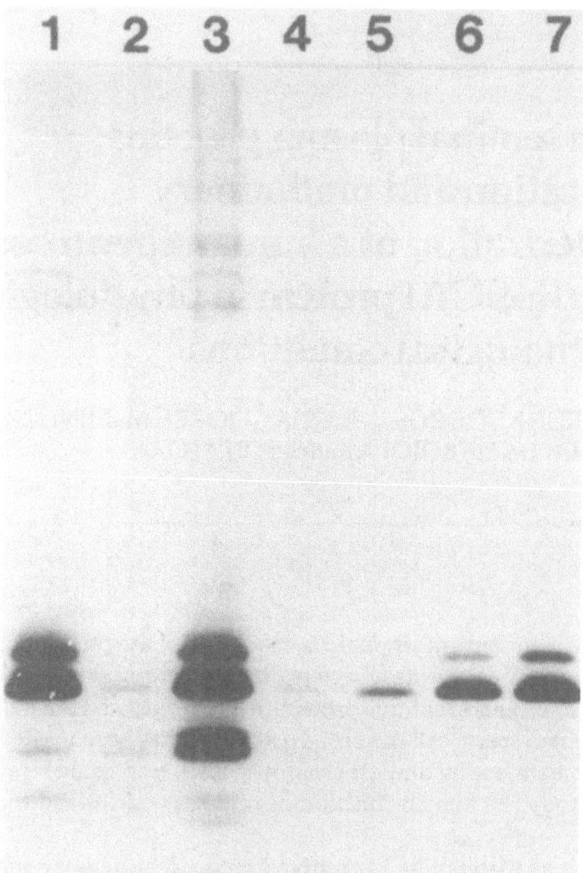

Figure 1 SDS-urea PAGE of ^{35}S-methionine labelled RSV-IV following immunoprecipitation with anti-RSV-IV antibodies in presence/absence of h-SP proteins

1. Labelled RSV-IV, following immunoprecipitation
2. as 1), but in presence of 5 μg of unlabelled native RSV-IV during the immunoprecipitation
3. Labelled *in vitro* translation products of total rat seminal vesicle mRNA
4. as 1), but with 625 μg of normal h-SP proteins during the immunoprecipitation
5. 6. and 7. 300 μg of normal, IHH and K h-SP proteins respectively present in the assay.
   SDS-urea PAGE analysis was performed in 15% polyacrylamide gels (acrylamide: bisacrylamide = 30% : 0.26%). The gels were prepared for fluorography according to a published procedure[4]

report a preliminary study on the detection in human seminal plasma of a protein (h-SCA) immunologically related to the major protein (RSV-IV) secreted by the epithelium of adult rat seminal vesicles[4]. In addition, by using a sensitive immunological assay specific for these proteins we have found that the expression of h-SCA gene(s) is seemingly under androgen control, testosterone not being the only requirement for h-SCA synthesis.

MATERIALS AND METHODS

Semen samples, obtained from healthy fertile volunteers and from individuals affected by Klinefelter's syndrome (KS) or idiopathic hypogonadotropic hypogonadism (IHH), were immediately diluted with one half volume of cold buffer containing 125 mmol/l NaCl, 5 mmol/l KCl, 1 mmol/l $MgSO_4$ 1 mmol/l EDTA, 40 mmol/l Tris·HCl, pH8, 3 mmol/l phenylmethyl-sulphonylfuoride (PMSF).

After centrifugation (25 000g, 5min, 4 °C) the supernatant fluid was dialysed at 4 °C against 20 mmol/l Tris·HCl pH8, 1 mmol/l EDTA, 3 mmol/l PMSF.

Preparation of ^{35}S-met labelled RSV-IV, SDS-urea PAGE analysis and competition RIA have been described elsewhere[4].

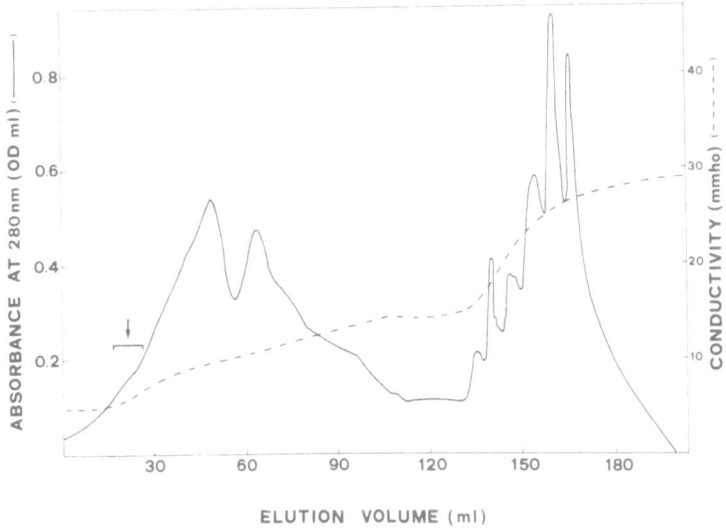

Figure 2   h-SP proteins fractionation by CM sepharose C50 chromatography

250 mg of h-SP proteins were loaded on a 0.9 cm × 10 cm column equilibrated in 0.1 mmol/l Na acetate pH 5.1. The elution was performed with an NaCl gradient in 0.1 mmol/l Na acetate pH 5.1. The proteins present in fractions 10–28 (see arrow), pooled and, concentrated by saturated ammonium sulphate precipitation, were further fractionated by gel filtration on Sephadex G 200. Few protein peaks were obtained; h-SCA fraction, eluting with MW 135 000, was detected by RIA.

RESULTS AND DISCUSSION

By using a competitive RIA with *in vitro* synthesized RSV-IV as radioactive antigen and specific rabbit anti-RSV-IV antibodies, we have detected h-SCA both in 1% Triton X100 washes of normal human spermatozoa (data not shown) and in normal human seminal plasma (Figure 1) h-SCA, present in human sperm, is a basic protein of molecular weight approximately 135 000 as demonstrated by chromatographic analysis (Figure 2) immunologically related to RSV-IV.

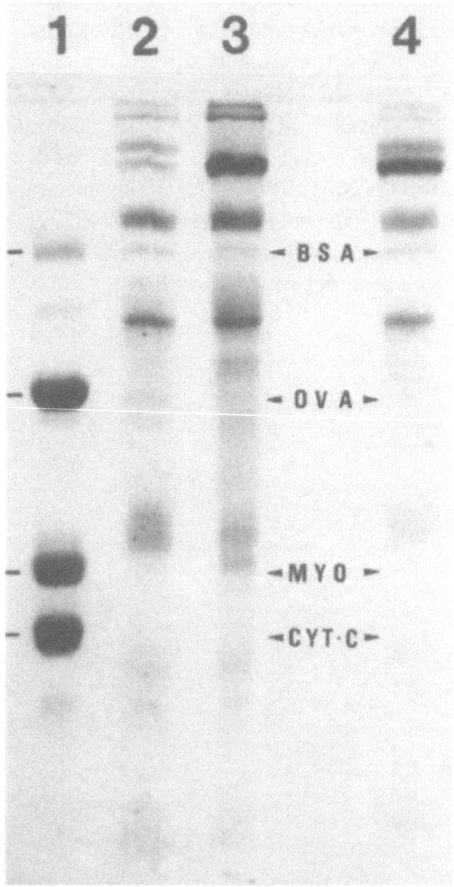

Figure 3 SDS-urea PAGE analysis of 100 μg of h-SP proteins from K(2), IHH (3) and normal (4) individuals following staining with Coomassie R250. In lane 1 the pattern of molecular weight markers is shown (BSA = 68 000; ovalbumin = 43 000; sperm whole myoglobulin = 17 200; Horse heart cytochrome C = 11 700). Experimental conditions for electrophoresis are described in Figure 1

SDS-urea PAGE analysis of seminal plasma from patients affected by KS have shown abnormal protein patterns (figure 3).

The immunoprecipitation of the RSV-IV complex in the presence of appropriate aliquots of different seminal plasma (normal and pathologic) has shown that 300 μg of normal h-SP proteins displace from anti-RSV-IV about 95% of RSV-IV, whereas the same amount of IHH or KS proteins 80–90% and 20–30%, respectively, as estimated by densitometric analysis of fluorograms (Figure 1).

All these data, taken together, suggest that h-SCA synthesis is apparently regulated by androgens, whereas in KS testosterone does not appear to be the essential requirement for a normal h-SCA synthesis.

References

1. Tauber, P. F., Zaneveld, L. J. D., Propping, D. and Schumacher, G. F. B. (1975). *J. Reprod. Fertil.*, **43**, 249–67
2. Guerin, J. F., Menezo, Y. and Ezyba, J. C. (1979). *Arch. Androl.*, **3**, 251–60
3. Blane, E. T. and Sensabaugh, G. F. (1978). *J. Forens. Sci.*, **23**, 717–29
4. Abrescia, P., Guardiola, J., Felsani, A. and Metafora, S. (1982). *Nucl. Acid Res.*, **10**, 1159–74

23
Antigenicity of sperm cells after freezing and thawing

M. PHILLIP, D. KLEINMAN, G. POTASHNIK and V. INSLER

INTRODUCTION

Seminal fluid contains antigens from the testis, epididymis, ejaculatory duct and the accessory glands[1]. These organs give rise to antigens differing in type and amount. The antigens in the seminal fluid can be divided into those that appear in the seminal plasma and those that are attached to the spermatozoal cell. The antigens attached to the spermatozoa are found in the head, mid-piece, main tail part and the end-piece.

In 1979, a review of a number of studies by Menge and Berman[1] reported that 7–17% of women with unexplained infertility had antibodies against male spermatozoa in their serum.

In 1973, Sherman[2] stated that even with the use of appropriate methods of freezing and thawing, spermatozoa undergo structural, physical and bio-chemical changes.

Alexander and Kay[3] claimed that the process of cryopreservation of spermatozoa causes surface changes thus decreasing the antigenicity of the spermatozoa. They also suggested that frozen semen samples may prove to be more effective for women with antisperm antibodies in their serum. If the assumption that in the process of cryopreservation there is a decrease in antigenicity of spermatozoa, then perhaps for the specific group of women with antibodies against spermatozoa, cryopreservation may be the treatment of choice for achieving fertilization.

In the work reported here, we have investigated whether any removal of antigens from the spermatozoal surface occurs during the process of freezing, preservation and thawing.

MATERIALS AND METHODS

All samples were taken from donors with blood group type O. Each donor's sample showed more than 60×10^6 cells/ml, initial motility above 60%, less than 40% abnormal morphological forms, and post-thaw motility above 40%. Each sample was divided into three parts: (1) fresh semen, (2) fresh semen mixed with glycerol to a final concentration of 7%, and (3) semen mixed with glycerol (final concentration of 7%) subjected to the freezing and thawing process. The freezing process was performed as described by Barkay[4]. All the frozen semen samples (part 3) were kept deeply frozen in liquid nitrogen at a temperature of $-196\,^\circ$C for 3–4 weeks. The presence of sperm antigens before and after freezing and thawing was investigated by means of the IPAMA (indirect immunoperoxidase antibody membrane antigen) test, the SIT (sperm immobilization test) and by separation of proteins by gel electrophoresis.

IPAMA

The sperm cells were washed three times in PBS. Drops of this suspension were placed on glass slides and dried at room temperature. The dried sperm cells were fixed and incubated with positive serum using human serum containing antibodies against spermatozoa. Rabbit immunoglobulin against human IgA/IgG diluted to 1:25 in PBS, were added and incubated for 45 minutes at $37\,^\circ$C in a humidified environment. Next, an antibody against rabbit IgG attached to peroxidase and diluted to a concentration of 1:20 in PBS, was added. The mixture was incubated for 45 minutes. After washing a colour reaction with substrate was performed. A positive reaction consisted of formation of a brown ring around the sperm cells[5]. By performing the IPAMA test on 20 different sperm cell samples and obtaining a positive reaction in all of them before and after freezing and thawing (Figure 1), the conclusion can be drawn that there is no significant removal of antigens from the surface membrane of sperm cells during the freezing and thawing process. This result does not exclude the possibility of partial removal of antigens, particularly those concerned with sperm immobilization. This possibility was examined by the SIT test in 10 different semen samples.

SIT (Sperm immobilization test)

This process is based on the evaluation of sperm motility in the presence of sperm containing specific antibodies against sperm cells. The antigen–antibody interaction activates the complement system, which in turn alters the permeability and integrity of the sperm cell. These changes manifest themselves by a reduction in serum motility. We observed complete

118

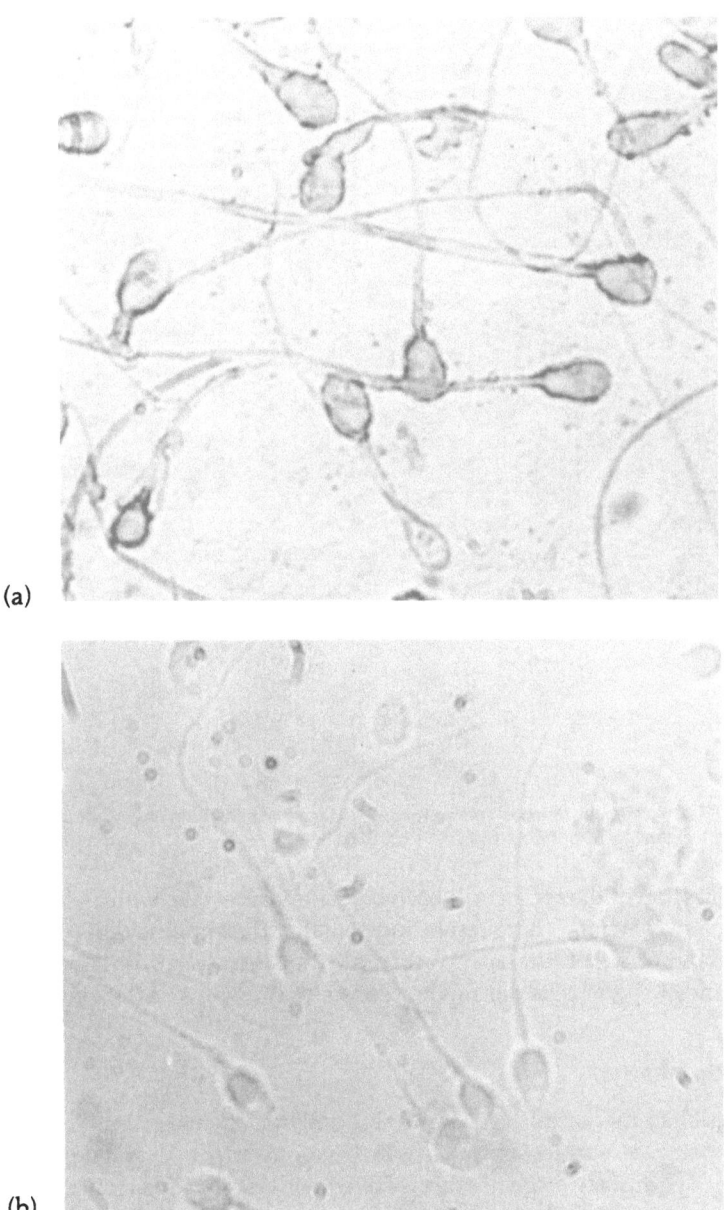

(a)

(b)

Figure 1 Photo micrograph of spermatozoa subjected to the indirect immunoperoxidase antibody membrane antigen (IPAMA) test. (a) Positive reaction showing the densely stained ring around spermatoa. (b) Negative reaction

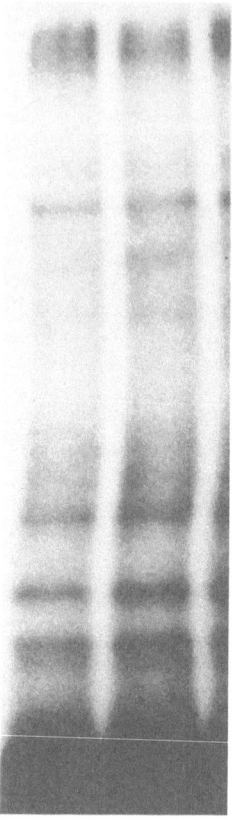

Figure 2   Gel electrophoresis of spermatozoal surface proteins showing eight bands with molecular weights corresponding to 17000–180 000

immobilization of the sperm cells both before and after (i.e. with and without) freezing and thawing. These results indicate that the antigens that participate in immobilization of the sperm cells are not removed from the surface membrane of sperm cells during the process of freezing and thawing.

Gel electrophoresis

The possibility that the process of freezing and thawing may result in removal of spermatozoal surface proteins was investigated in 10 different semen samples. The surface proteins were labelled with radioactive iodine and then separated using gel electrophoresis. Very similar separation strips were obtained before freezing and after thawing. Both showed eight different bands with molecular weights of 180 000, 105 000, 84 000, 74 000, 37 000, 30 000, 25 000 and 17 000 (Figure 2).

DISCUSSION

The present study, using three different methods, indicates that the process of freezing, cryopreservation and thawing of spermatozoa does not result in a significant removal of antigens from the surface of the sperm cells.

Hence this study does not support the suggestion of Alexander[3] that, in cases of immunological incompatibility between spermatozoa and cervical mucus, it would be possible to overcome the couples' infertility by freezing, preservation and thawing of the husband's spermatozoa.

References

1. Menge, A. C. and Berman, S. J. (1979). Immunologic Infertility. *Clin. Obstet. Gynecol.*, **22**, 231
2. Sherman, J. K. (1973). Synopsis of the use of frozen human semen since 1964. State of the art of human semen banking. *Fertil. Steril.*, **2**, 397
3. Alexander, N. J. (1977). Antigenicity of frozen and fresh spermatozoa. *Fertil. Steril.*, **28**, 1234
4. Barkay, J., Zuckerman, H. and Heiman, ?. (1974). A new practical method of freezing and storing human sperm and a preliminary report in its use. *Fertil. Steril.*, **25**, 399
5. Geno, G., McCloud, C. J. and Chambers, R. W. (1976). Immunoperoxidase technique for detection of antibodies to human cytomegalovirus. *J. Clin. Microbiol.*, **3**, 364–72

.

24
A radioimmunoassay for antisperm antibodies using ^{125}I-labelled protein A

D. CANNON, G. MCKENNA, J. HARNEY, J. BARRON,
B. M. COUGHLAN and D. POWELL

INTRODUCTION

Autoimmunity to spermatozoa may be an important cause of infertility. However, many current methods for the estimation of antisperm antibody activity lack reliability, specificity and sensitivity. This paper reports the use of ^{125}I-labelled Protein A (^{125}I-PA) from *Staphylococcus aureus* as a specific and sensitive immunological probe to detect antisperm-antibody activity in male sera. The characteristic biological property of protein A is its ability to interact with a variety of IgG molecules. Humoral antisperm antibodies in males are predominantly of the IgG class[1], and, therefore, react with protein A. As the interaction takes place via the Fc region of IgG[2], the antigen-binding region is free to form antibody–antigen complexes. The selectivity of protein A makes this reagent a versatile tool with many potential applications to immunology.

MATERIAL AND METHODS

Serum was obtained from nine males whose semen contained agglutinated spermatozoa in consecutive samples, from thirteen males with antisperm positive sera (WHO, Aarhus, Denmark) and from 12 control males (eight with proven fertility).

Normal volunteer semen was washed twice with PBS buffer (containing 0.3% BSA and 0.2% azide), centrifuged (800 g) for 10 min, and the supernatant replaced with buffer to give a count of 60×10^6/ml. The washed sample was stored at 4 °C.

A 50 µl aliquot of serially diluted serum from patients or controls was mixed with a 50 µl aliquot of stored sperm suspension (3×10^6) in a polystyrene tube, covered and placed in a waterbath at 37 °C for 3 hours. After incubation, 500 µl buffer was added, mixed and the tubes centrifuged. The supernatant was decanted. 100 µl (20 000 c.p.m.) ^{125}I-protein A (Amersham International Ltd., UK) was added to the pellet, mixed and further incubated at 37 °C for 1.5 hours. The suspension was then washed with 1 ml buffer, centrifuged and the supernatant decanted. Non-specific binding was estimated by incubation of spermatozoa and ^{125}I-protein A without serum. Sensitivity was optimized by varying incubation times and temperatures of sperm/serum mixture (Figure 1) and sperm/^{125}I-protein A mixture (Figure 2).

RESULTS AND DISCUSSION

Maximum sensitivity was achieved by incubation of sperm/serum mixture for 3 hours at 37 °C, and sperm/^{125}I-protein A for 1.5 hours at 37 °C (Figures 1 and 2). Serum from all patients caused a dilution-dependent binding of ^{125}I-protein A to spermatozoa (Figure 3). No control serum caused ^{125}I-protein A binding. Non-specific binding was less than 5%. The dilution curves of

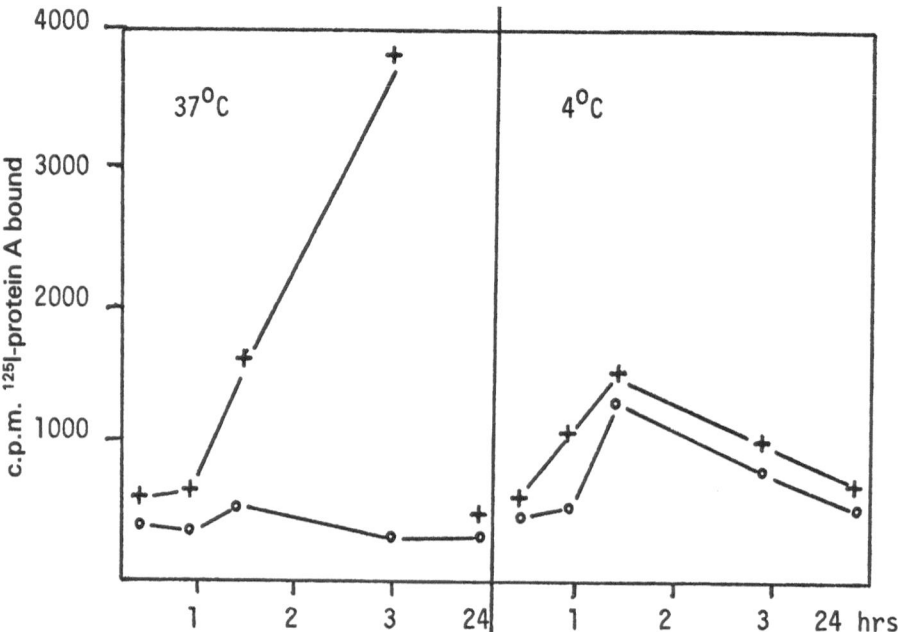

Figure 1 Binding of ^{125}I-protein A to sperm (1.5 h, 37 °C) after varying preincubation times at 37 °C and 4 °C with control (o—o) or patient's (+ — +) serum

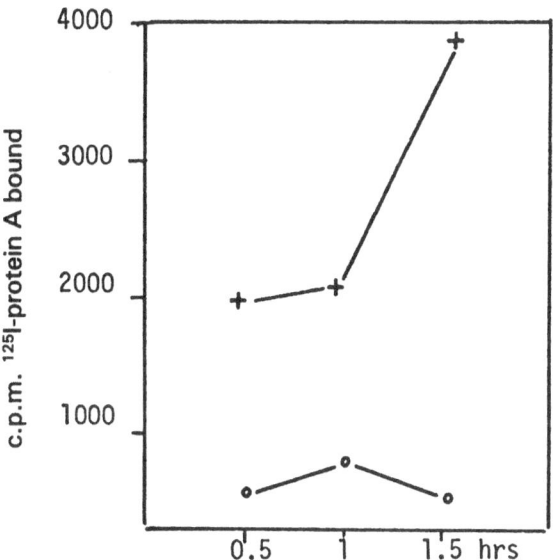

Figure 2 Rate of binding of ¹²⁵I-protein A to sperm pellet following preincubation (3 h, 37 °C) with control (o—o) or patient's (+ — +) serum

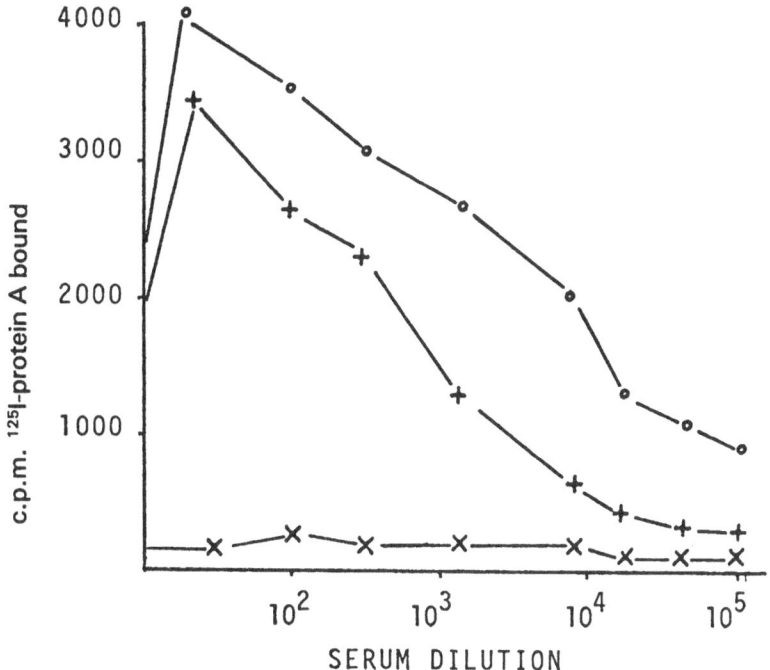

Figure 3 Dilution curves for WHO sera 29 (+), 30 (o) and a control (X)

patients sera displayed characteristic responses; at serum dilutions of 1/8, or higher in some cases ^{125}I-protein A binding was inhibited. Subsequent dilutions followed a linear pattern (Figure 3). A comparison of antibody titres was obtained using gelatine agglutination test (GAT), the tray agglutination test (TAT) and the ^{125}I-protein A assay and is shown in Table 1.

Table 1   A comparison of the antibody titres obtained with the GAT, TAT and ^{125}I-protein A assay for some of the WHO sera. R. R. and G. S. were patients attending an infertility clinic at the Mater Hospital

WHO number	GAT titre	TAT titre	^{125}I-protein A assay titre
29	512	1024	32 000
30	512	2048	128 000
31	1024	4096	32 000
32	512	1024	64 000
95	256	256	32 000
97	128	128	128 000
98	32	32	64 000
R. R.	512	1024	16 000
G. S.	512	1024	16 000

CONCLUSION

The ^{125}I-protein A assay offers many advantages:

(1)   It does not require fresh motile sperm,
(2)   Non-specific binding is always low,
(3)   Antibodies additional to agglutinating antibodies are detected,
(4)   Sensitivity is much greater (at least by 10^2) than existing serological methods.

ACKNOWLEDGEMENTS

I wish to acknowledge the co-operation of Dr T. Hjort, University of Aarhus, Denmark, who supplied a selection of samples and results of various agglutination tests.

References

1. Ingerslav, H. J., Hjort, T. and Linnet, L. (1979). Immunoglobulin classes of human sperm antibodies; Immunoaffinity chromatographic analysis with special attention to agglutinating and immobilizing activity of IgG and IgM. *J. Clin. Lab. Immunol.*, 2, 239
2. Forsgren, A. and Sjoquist, J. (1966). 'Protein A' from *Staphylococcus aureus*. 1. Pseudo-immune reaction with human γ-globulin. *J. Immunol.*, 97, 822

25
Human cervical response to artificial insemination

I. J. PANDYA and J. COHEN

INTRODUCTION

The response of the female tract to the presence of male antigens is complex and poorly understood. This immunological encounter is central to the normal reproductive process. Austin[1] investigated the rabbit vaginal and uterine response to semen and found phagocytosis; Phillips and Mahler[2] compared the rabbit vaginal response to whole semen and to sperm-free seminal plasma. They found phagocytes in both cases, suggesting that a leukocytic response can be triggered by some agent in semen other than spermatozoa. Tyler[3] however, investigated the rabbit cervical response to sperm-free seminal plasma and found that there was little leukocytic reaction compared with the enormous response to whole semen. He concluded that leukocytosis is triggered by spermatozoa and not by seminal plasma or copulation. This present study was designed to determine whether a similar response could be demonstrated in humans, and whether it was elicited by spermatozoa or by other male antigens.

MATERIALS AND METHODS

Women volunteers of apparently normal fertility were recruited from the Artificial Insemination Clinic. Insemination was timed to coincide with ovulation as judged by cervical mucus. A cusco speculum, lubricated with warm water, was used to get an unobstructed view of the cervix. The woman was judged to be within 1 day of ovulation if our modified Insler score was ≥ 6 out of 12.

The tests were not performed if there was an erosion or inflammation. The ectocervix was cleaned gently twice with 0.9% saline using sterile gauze swabs.

Artificial insemination was carried out by introducing 0.5 ml of semen into the mucus of the external cervical os, directly from a polythene 'straw'. The cervix was sampled by drawing the edge of a wooden Ayre spatula about 1 cm across the moist tissue surface and then across a clean microscope slide. Smears were fixed immediately in alcohol (64 OP) for at least 30 minutes and stained automatically by the Papanicolaou[4] technique. Leukocytes and squamous cells were counted using bright field illumination, Neofluar 40 objective, 0.65 NA (×480 total magnification). Results were expressed as a ratio: leukocytes per hundred squamous cells. Because nearly all leukocytes were polymorphonuclear neutrophils, no further analysis was performed.

Four different sites of the cervix were chosen for smears at different times, to check the response to the smearing as well as to the insemination; and to ascertain whether leukocytes were already present or were being elicited by the smearing.

Seminal plasma containing spermatozoa was obtained from donors or husbands, while seminal plasma without spermatozoa was obtained from azoospermic husbands or vasectomized volunteers. Samples were mixed with egg yolk and buffer and were frozen and stored at −196 °C in liquid nitrogen. Semen was thawed by leaving straws at room temperature for about 5 minutes. Routine microscopic assessment before insemination was carried out to exclude any obvious bacterial infection.

The first group of women was artifically inseminated with 0.5 ml frozen–thawed semen, the second group with 0.5 ml fresh semen (within 2 h of ejaculation), the third group with 0.5 ml frozen sperm-free seminal plasma and the fourth group with 0.5 ml fresh sperm-free seminal plasma. Smears were taken at 15 min before and just before the insemination. As there was no significant difference between these smears for the whole series, the mean of the two smears was taken as a base line. Then smears were taken at 15 min, 4 h and 24 h post-insemination.

RESULTS

Thirty out of 100 women agreed to co-operate. Two patients were unable to attend the clinic for the 24 h post-insemination smears, and one could not attend for the 4 h and 24 h post-insemination smears. Smears from three patients had to be discarded due to slight bleeding at the site of the smear.

Three women had had sexual intercourse with their oligozoospermic husbands less than 24 h before insemination; their pre-insemination smears showed the presence of a large number of leukocytes. Two other women, who had had sexual intercourse with their oligozoospermic husbands more than 24 hours before insemination, showed the presence of a few leukocytes. The smears from one woman who had sexual intercourse with her severely oligo-zoospermic husband within 24 h before insemination showed the presence of a very few leukocytes.

The first two groups of women (who were inseminated with frozen-thawed or fresh semen), reacted to it by a marked cervical leukocytosis. The response was variable between women. In cases of all women but one who had had sexual intercourse before insemination, the initial smears showed the presence of a large number of leukocytes. The number rose slightly at $+15$ min, but dropped markedly by 4 h and rose again within 24 h (Figure 1). All women who did not have sexual intercourse for at least 60 h before insemination, showed the presence of a very few leukocytes in the first smear. The number rose slightly by 15 min, rose very markedly by 4 h, and fell slightly by 24 h (Figure 1).

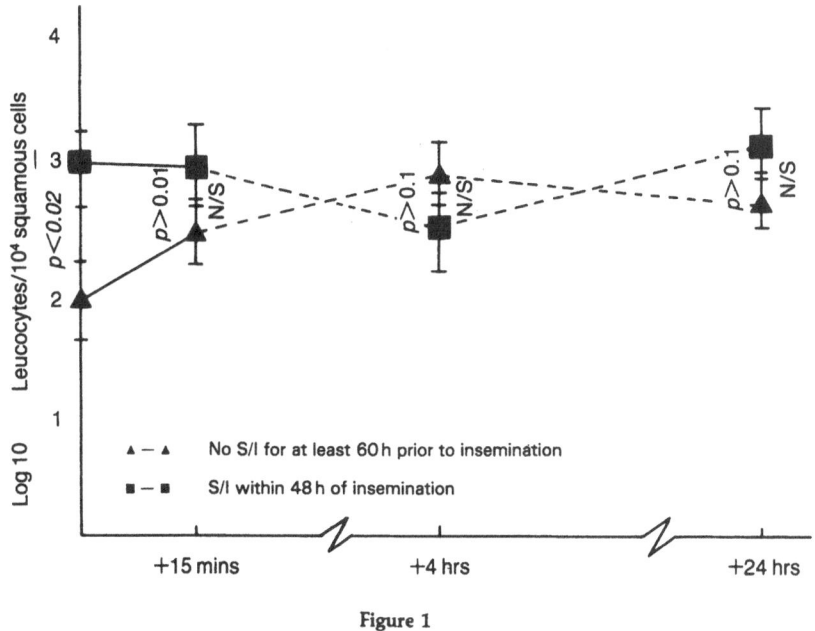

Figure 1

Groups 3 and 4, who were inseminated with either frozen–thawed or fresh sperm-free seminal plasma, showed *no* significant leukocytosis (Figure 2).

Two patients actually became pregnant by the monitored insemination, while one became pregnant during a subsequent cycle.

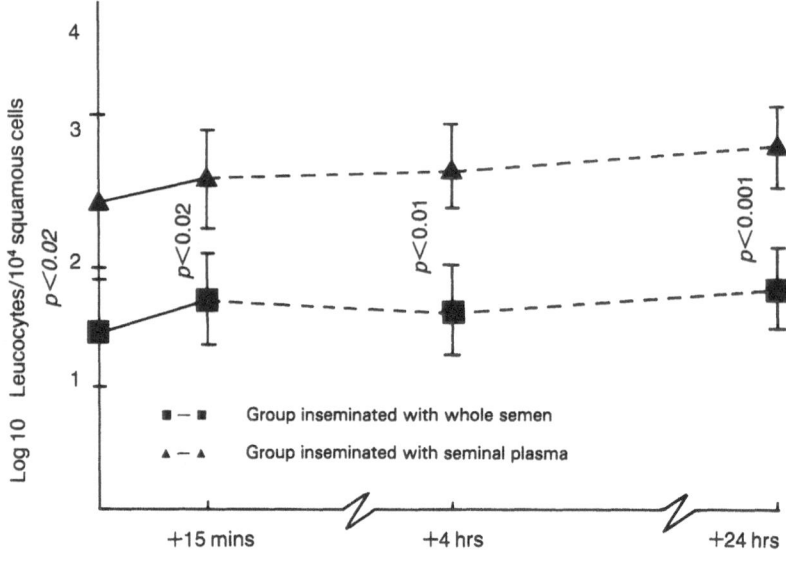

Figure 2

DISCUSSION

There was clear and consistent evidence of leukocytosis in the cervix of women who had had sexual intercourse with oligozoospermic husbands prior to insemination. Artificial insemination without spermatozoa showed no reaction, but with spermatozoa showed a strong reaction in all women tested. This shows that the reaction is evoked by spermatozoa and that other seminal components (including egg yolk or buffer) have little if any effect.

That this leukocytosis is physioligical is convincingly justified by the initiation of pregnancies by the observed AIDs. This is consistent with the conclusion of Taylor[5] that leukocytosis does not form any barrier to effective spermatozoa.

There is a very important clinical corollary to this establishment of post-coital leukocytosis as a normal physiological reaction. The finding of leukocytes in cervical smears should not, in future, be equated with patho-logical cervicitis; if spermatozoa are present as well, the leukocytes are only evidence of this newly-discovered part of the normal human coital physiology.

ACKNOWLEDGEMENT

Our thanks to Professor J. R. Newton for his facilities and encouragement.

References

1. Austin, C. R. (1976). Fate of spermatozoa in the female genital tract and the problem of induction of local anti-sperm immunity in women. Proceedings of the 3rd *International Symposium on the Immunology of Reproduction.* pp. 63–80 (Varna, Bulgaria (Copenhagen: Scripter)
2. Phillips, D. M. and Mahler, S. (1975). Migration of leucocytes and phagocytosis in rabbit vagina. *J. Cell Biol.,* **67,** 334a
3. Tyler, K. R. (1977). Histological changes in the cervix of the rabbit after coitus. *J. Reprod. Fertil.,* 341–45
4. Papanicolaou, R. (1942). Technique for staining smears. *J. Lab. Clin. Med.,* **26,** 1200
5. Taylor, N. J. (1982). Investigation of sperm-induced cervical leucocytosis by a double mating study in rabbits. *J. Reprod. Fertil.,* **66,** 157–60

Section 4

Medical Treatment of the Infertile Male

26
Kallman's syndrome – sustained spermatogenesis three years after cessation of treatment

A. I. TRAUB, A. B. ATKINSON and W. THOMPSON

INTRODUCTION

Isolated gonadotropin deficiency (IGD) is a rare condition leading to a deficiency in LH and FSH production, and a subsequent underproduction of testosterone in the male and oestrogen in the female[1]. When these defects are associated with anosmia it is known as Kallman's syndrome[2]. The absence of the gonadotropins, FSH and LH, results in failure of sexual maturation, and the normal process of puberty is not completed. The gonadotropin deficiency is usually bihormonal, and although virilization and fertility can be achieved using gonadotropin therapy, these are temporary and relapse occurs with cessation of treatment. We describe a case of Kallman's syndrome in whom virilization, sexual maturation, a normal semen analysis and fertility were achieved using replacement therapy. This patient has remained virilized with normal semen analysis and testosterone levels for 3 years after cessation of all treatment.

PATIENT AND INVESTIGATIONS

The patient presented at age 25 with a history of primary infertility. He also spontaneously complained that his voice was high-pitched and that he did not need to shave, although his libido was normal and he denied coital problems. On further questioning he admitted to never having had a sense of smell. A paternal uncle, now dead, also had anosmia. There was nothing else of note in his medical or family history.

On examination he was of average height and build with a slight cranio-facial asymmetry. There was no facial hair but pubic hair was normally developed. The penis was normal but small; the testes were both palpable in the scrotum and were also small. Anosmia was confirmed using nitrobenzene, camphor and oil of cloves.

Basal serum hormone levels were total thyroxine (TT4) 78 nmol/l (50–150), TSH 1.0 mu/l (< 5), ACTH 48.0 (< 85 ng/ml), prolactin 133 mu/l (< 300), growth hormone 0.9 mu/l (< 5), FSH 0.4 mu/l (0.2–6.0), LH 3.6 mu/l (0.4–10) and testosterone 3.4 nmol/l (9.5–24.5). The gonadotropins were thus inappropriately low for the sex steroid levels. An X-ray of the pituitary fossa was normal. Three semen analyses revealed azoospermia, with volumes of 0.5 ml.

Treatment was initiated with oral mesterolone (Proviron) 50 mg daily for 6 months, at the end of which time no change had occurred in his voice or beard growth. A repeat semen analysis again showed azoospermia; FSH at this time remained low – FSH 0.5 mu/l, LH 3.6 mu/l and testosterone 5.9 mnol/l. Replacement therapy was then changed to testosterone propionate 250 mg intramuscularly at 2 weekly intervals. After a further 6 months, the patient had experienced no significant improvement. Treatment was stopped for 6 months at the patient's request and, at the end of this period, further investigation showed FSH 1.7 mu/l, LH 4.0 mu/l and testosterone 7.4 nmol/l. There was still no improvement in his voice or facial hair but semen analysis for the first time showed motile sperm in small amounts (total count 4.5 million/ml with 15% motility; volume 0.5 ml).

Gonadotropin therapy was commenced using menotrophin (Pergonal), two ampoules (75 IU of hCG and hMG) with Pregnyl (hCG) 3000 IU three times per week intramuscularly. After 3 months the patient's voice had deepened and he was shaving occasionally: the sperm count had risen to 30×10^6/ml with 50% motility; 4 weeks later his sperm count was 45×10^6/ml, but the volume remained low at 0.5 ml. His therapy was changed to Pregnyl 5000 IU twice per week, and continued for 3 months, after which time, the sperm count was 90×10^6/ml, (total volume 0.5 ml), the voice had broken and he needed to shave on alternate days. All treatment was then stopped at his request. Five months later his wife had conceived, at which time his sperm count was 30×10^6/ml, with 50% motility (total volume 0.8 ml). The pregnancy progressed normally and a healthy female infant was born at term. The patient did not attend for follow-up for a further year at which time he still needed to shave daily and his voice was normal. Serum FSH was 2.6 mu/l, LH was 6.5 mu/l and testosterone was 19 nmol/l. Sperm count was 65×10^6/ml, with 55% motility and volume 0.8 ml. One year later, semen analysis was entirely normal and most recently, after 3 years the semen volume was 2.8 ml with a count of 75×10^6/ml and 50% motility. Serum testosterone was normal, 17.4 nmol/l and FSH 2.2 mu/l, LH 7.7 mu/l.

DISCUSSION

The differential diagnosis of delayed puberty[1] with low gonadotropin levels lies between constitutionally delayed puberty and hypogonadotrophic hypogonadism. Although various tests have been put forward as aids to the diagnosis none are foolproof[1,3-6]. However, in the case under discussion there were two main arguments for a diagnosis of isolated gonadotropin deficiency, namely the patient's age and the associated anosmia[2].

Having made a diagnosis of Kallman's syndrome, it was of interest that testosterone therapy produced only very minor alterations in the secondary sexual characteristics of the patient. This was a surprising aspect of the case and we consider it possible that the patient had not been compliant. Nevertheless, during the period of testosterone therapy, sperm, albeit in the severely oligozoospermic range, appeared in the ejaculate. The reasons for this are not immediately obvious. However, it is known that in the rat, testosterone alone is capable of maintaining spermatogenesis after hypophysectomy. One possibility is that if the hormone is present in a high enough concentration it may act without the required amplification of its action by FSH-induced production of androgen-binding protein (ABP), while the other possibility is that small amounts of endogeneous FSH were already producing some ABP[8]. A number of similar cases have been documented in the older literature[9,10] but these were prior to the development of reliable assays for serum gonadotropins.

The effect of menotrophin and hCG was to produce a normal sperm count after 3 months, an interval in keeping with the length of time required for sperm maturation. Normally gonadotropin treatment would be continued until pregnancy occurred but, fortunately in this case, despite cessation of treatment at the patient's request, pregnancy was achieved 5 months later.

This case is thus of particular note not only because a minor degree of spermatogenesis occurred with testosterone therapy alone but because spermatogenesis remained normal 3 years after stopping all treatment. A number of cases have been reported in which spermatogenesis has been maintained for varying intervals while treatment was maintained, but not thereafter[1,11,12]. Had our patient not had anosmia the maintenance of secondary sexual characteristics and of spermatogenesis would probably have led to the diagnosis of an extreme case of constitutional delay of puberty. To our knowledge there has, previous to the case under discussion, been no documented report of Kallman's syndrome where normal spermatogenesis continued after treatment was stopped.

Our hypothesis in the present case of established Kallman's syndrome is that the patient exhibited a milder form of gonadotropin deficiency, a disorder known to be heterogeneous in its manifestations, with partial bihormonal deficiency of LH and FSH. The small amounts of endogenous LH and FSH were insufficient to induce puberty, spermatogenesis or normal secondary sexual characteristics. However, when these were induced by therapy the low levels of endogenous gonadotropin have been sufficient to maintain normal sexual function for 3 years without therapy. The present case would suggest that, in man, more gonadotropin is needed to induce puberty than to maintain sexual potency.

References

1. Rabinowitz, D. and Spitz, I. M. (1975). Isolated gonadotropin deficiency and related disorders. *Isr. J. Med. Sci.*, 11, 1011–78
2. Kallman, F. J., Schoenfeld, W. A. and Barrera, S. E. (1944). The genetic aspects of primary eunuchoidism. *Am. J. Metal. Defic.*, 68, 203
3. Girard, J., Baumann, J. B. and Ruch, W. (1980). Diagnostic possibilities in delayed puberty. In Cacciari, E. and Prader, A. (eds.) *Serono Symposium No. 36, Pathophysiology of Puberty.* p. 223 (London, New York: Academic Press)
4. Troen, P. and Oshima, H. (1981). The Testis. In Felig, P., Baxter, J. D., Broadus, A. C. and Frohman, L. A. (eds.) *Endocrinology and Metabolism.* p. 639. (New York: McGraw Hill)
5. Hamilton, C. R., Henkin, R. I., Weir, G. and Kliman, B. (1973). Olfactory status and response to clomiphene in male gonadotropin deficiency. *Ann. Intern. Med.*, 78, 47
6. Spitz, I. M., Hirsch, H. J. and Trestian, S. (1983). The prolactin response to thyrotropin-releasing hormone differentiates isolated gonadotropin deficiency from delayed puberty. *N. Engl. J. Med.*, 308, 575
7. Prader, A. (1975). Disorders of Puberty. *Clin. Endocrinol. Metab.*, 4, 143
8. Rabin, D. and McKenna, T. J. (1982). The regulation of gonadotropin secretion in males. In Rabin, D. and McKenna, T. J. (eds.) *Clinical Endocrinology and Metabolism, Principles and Practice.* p. 577. (New York: Grune and Stratton)
9. Kinsell, L. W. (1947). Spermatogenesis in a 'pan-hypopituitary' eunuchoid, as the result of testosterone therapy. *J. Clin. Endocrinol.*, 7, 781
10. Werner, S. C. (1951). Spermatogenesis and apparent fertility in a eunuchoid male in the eleventh year of androgen therapy. *J. Clin. Endocrinol. Metab.*, 11, 612
11. Martin, F. I. R. (1967). The stimulation and prolonged maintenance of spermatogenesis in a patient with hypogonadotrophic hypogonadism. *J. Endocrinol.*, 38, 431
12. Granville, G. E. (1970). Successful gonadotropin therapy of infertility in a hypopituitary man. *Arch. Intern. Med.*, 125, 1041

27
Effects of testosterone undecanoate on semen quality and sexual behaviour

D. DA RUGNA and J. SAASTAMOINEN

INTRODUCTION

Orally administered testosterone is almost ineffective because of its premature inactivation by the liver. Intramuscular administration and implantation are unfavourable for practical reasons. The fatty acid ester of the androgen, testosterone undecanoate (TU), has been shown to be an orally effective preparation, resulting in an increase[1] of plasma T, a decrease of elevated gonadotropin concentrations[1] and improvement in sexual behaviour[2].

PATIENTS AND METHODS

185 men from primary (seldom secondary) infertile couples who showed, on two semen analyses at least one or more abnormal findings according to Eliasson[3] classification were evaluated after TU-treatment. The age of the patients varied between 22–45 y, average 31.6 y. Volume, sperm count, motility and morphology before treatment were compared with the findings generally 10 weeks after treatment. The treatment was rated as successful (+), if with reference to the scheme of Eliasson a higher level of quality was obtained; as worsening (−), if there was a decrease to a lower level or as unchanged (=), if the quality remained the same. The following dosages were applied:

2 × daily 40 mg for 60 days (4800 mg total):	135 patients
3 × daily 40 mg for 40 days (4800 mg) total):	13 patients
2 × daily 40 mg for 90 days (7200 mg total):	7 patients
3 × daily 40 mg for 60 days (7200 total):	24 patients
other doses (total 2400–2 × 7200 mg):	6 patients

RESULTS

Semen quality

The semen *volume*, estimated over the whole group, did not show an improvement (16% +, 12% −, 72% =). The sperm *count* was also not improved (15% +, 12% −, 73% =). The relatively low dose used in the majority of the cases gave an increase in only 13% and a decrease in 15%.

The best results were obtained in regard of *motility*. Taken together, 41% of the cases improved. Analysing these effects by the binomial distribution, the positive results are significant ($p<0.02$). Comparison of the various dosages shows no important differences.

Table 1   Sperm motility

Dosage	Number of patients	Results +	−	=
2×40 mg for 60 d (Total 4800 mg)	134	51 (38%)	24 (18%)	59 (44%)
3×40 mg for 40 d (Total 4800 mg)	13	6	1	6
2×40 mg for 90 d (Total 7200 mg)	6	2	2	2
3×40 mg for 60 d (Total 7200 mg)	24	12	2	10
Other doses	6	4	1	1
Total	183	75 (41%)	30 (16%)	78 (43%)

Concerning *morphology* the same conclusion can be drawn as for volume and count: on the whole no success (13% +, 9% −, 78% =).

Pregnancies

The number of pregnancies obtained was 26, i.e. 14% of the cases treated. Referring to the different dosages, the distribution is as follows:

2×40 mg (total of 4800 mg): 19 out of 135 (14%); 3×40 mg (total of 1 out of 13)

2×40 mg (total of 7200 mg): 4 out of 7; and 3×40 mg (total of 7200 mg) 2 out of 24.

The rate of 14% pregnancies cannot be interpreted as a therapeutic effect, because similar fertility rates may be expected without treatment, and in some cases the wives were treated at the same time.

EFFECTS ON SEXUAL BEHAVIOUR

Fourteen patients with various degrees of impotence were treated and analysed. The age varied from 23 to 61 years, the mean age being 42.6 y. The dosage was usually 40 mg twice or three times daily for 20–30 days. Partial success was obtained in eight patients, i.e. improved ability for intercourse, prolonged and intensified erection. Only one case showed a definite change to normal behaviour.

Summing up, the effect of TU on sexual behaviour must be judged as unsatisfactory, although the results were somewhat better than those obtained earlier using a different androgen.

References

1. Mies, R. and Krempl, S. (1980). Die Wirkung von Testosteronundecanoat beim männlichen Hypogonadismus. *Med. Welt.*, **31**, 619
2. Luisi, M. and Franchi, F. (1980). Double-blind group comparative study of testosterone undecanoate and Mesterolone in hypogonadal male patients. *J. Endocrinol. Invest.*, **3**, 305
3. Eliasson, R. (1981). Analysis of semen. In Burger, H. and de Kretser, D. (eds.). *The Testis*, p. 381. (New York: Raven Press)

28
Tamoxifen in the treatment of reduced
semen quality: Preliminary results

E. W. JECHT, C. HIRSCHHÄUSER and W. KRAUSE

The effect of tamoxifen (T) on semen quality has been the subject of several reports[1-6]. An increase in sperm density was seen in most studies[1,3-6], while sperm motility improved in some studies[4,6] and did not in others[1,2,5]. For sperm morphology, no detailed analysis has been presented by any of the studies published so far. According to Schill and Landthaler[4], T did not affect sperm morphology, and Buvat et al.[5] reported no change in the percentage of abnormal forms.

Eighty patients were treated with tamoxifen (10 mg twice daily) for 3–5 months. An increase of sperm density was observed 3–5 months following the onset of treatment; this increase was, however, statistically not significant.

Twenty-six of the 80 patients were further analysed with regard to their hormonal concentrations. Only patients having a basal FSH concentration of 10 mIU/ml or less were included. There was a clear increase in the concentration of LH, FSH, testosterone, and E_2 as well as in sperm density 3 months after the initiation of the treatment with tamoxifen. No change was seen in the concentration of prolactin nor in sperm motility (Figures 1 and 2).

Examination of sperm morphology demonstrated no significant alteration in the percentage of abnormal forms in 33 patients treated with T for 3 months. However, the detailed analysis of the various abnormal forms demonstrated an increase in the percentage of sperms with anomalies of neck and midpiece (Figure 3) and a decrease of round heads (Figure 4).

Our results confirm those of the previous studies with regard to sperm density and endocrine parameters. The absence of an improvement in sperm motility agrees with the results of some investigators[1,2,5] and disagrees with

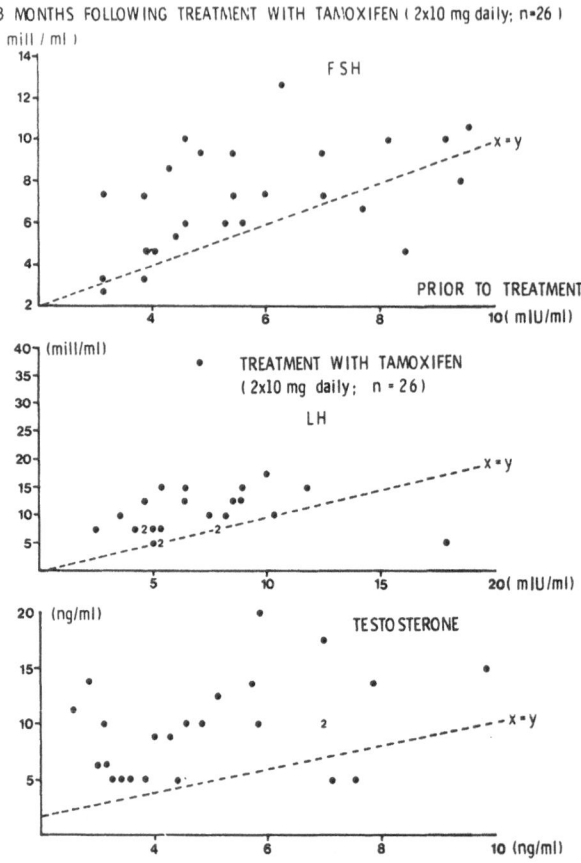

Figure 1 Concentrations of FSH, LH and testosterone prior to, and 3 months following, treatment with tamoxifen (2×10 mg/day)

those of others[4,6]. This difference may be due to the subjective assessment of sperm motility. The lack of a change in the concentration of prolactin is not surprising; still, no data have so far been published for this hormone during treatment with T[7].

We could confirm that T does not affect the percentage of abnormal forms. The changes seen in the percentages of round heads and of sperms with anomalies of neck and midpiece indicate, however, that T may have an effect on sperm morphology. Such an effect may not manifest itself in the percentage of abnormal forms due to the balancing increase of one abnormal form and the decrease of another.

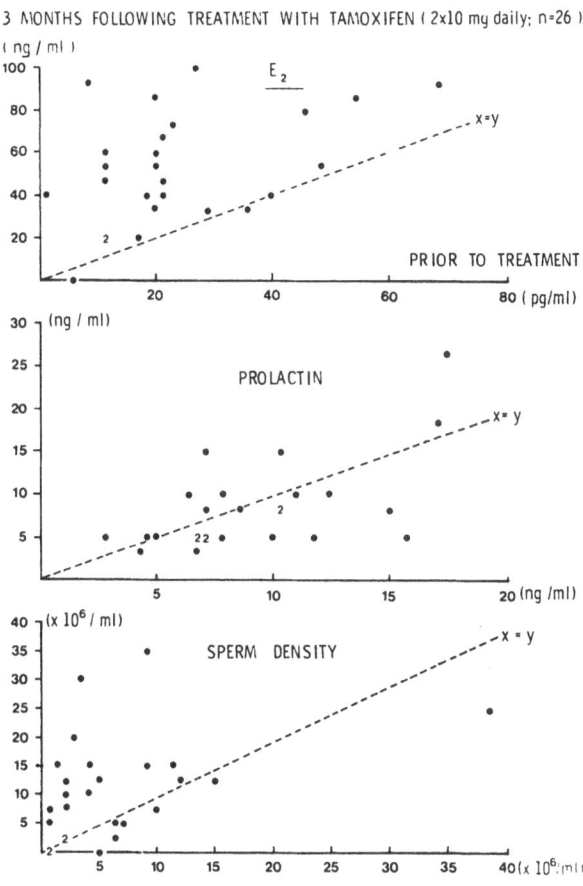

Figure 2 Concentrations of oestradiol, prolactin, and spermatozoa prior to, and 3 months following, treatment with tamoxifen (2 × 20 mg/day)

References

1. Comhaire, F. (1976). Treatment of oligospermia with tamoxifen. *Int. J. Fertil.*, **21**, 232
2. Willis, K.J., London, D.R., Bevis, M.A., Butt, W.R., Lynch, S.S. and Holder, G. (1977). Hormonal effects of tamoxifen in oligospermic men. *J. Endocrinol.*, **73**, 171
3. Vermeulen, A. and Comhaire, F. (1978). Hormonal effects of an antiestrogen, tamoxifen, in normal and oligospermic men. *Fertil. Steril.*, **29**, 320
4. Schill, W.-B. and Landthaler, M. (1980). Tamoxifen treatment of oligozoospermia. *Andrologia*, **12**, 546
5. Buvat, J., Gauthier, A., Ardaens, K., Buvat-Herbaut, M. and Lemaire, A. (1982). Effets du Tamoxifen sur les hormones et le sperme de 80 sujets oligospermiques et asthénospermiques. *J. Gynecol. Obstet. Biol. Repr.*, **11**, 407

6. Schieber, K. and Bartsch, G. (1982). Tamoxifen treatment in oligospermia. *Congress of the European Association of Urology*, 12–15 May, Vienna
7. Comhaire, F.H. (1982). Treatment of male infertility, Bain, J., Schill, W.-B. and Schwarzstein, L. (eds.) *Tamoxifen*. p. 45 (Berlin, Heidelberg, New York: Springer)

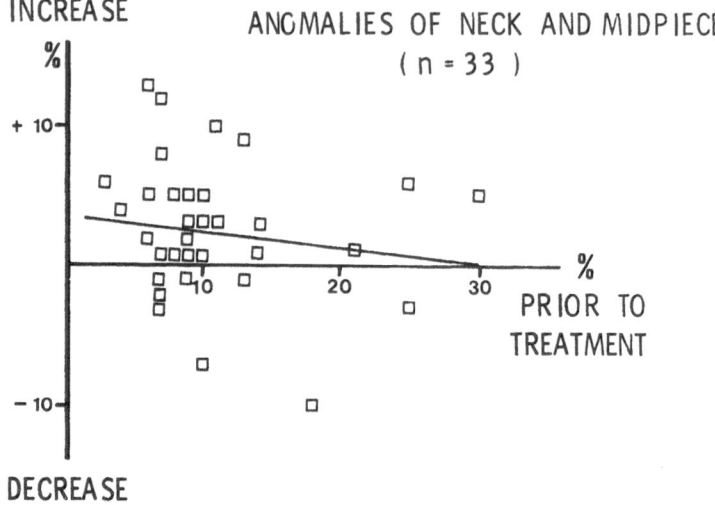

Figure 3 Effect of treatment with tamoxifen for 3 months (2×10 mg/day) on the percentage of spermatozoa with anomalies of neck and midpiece

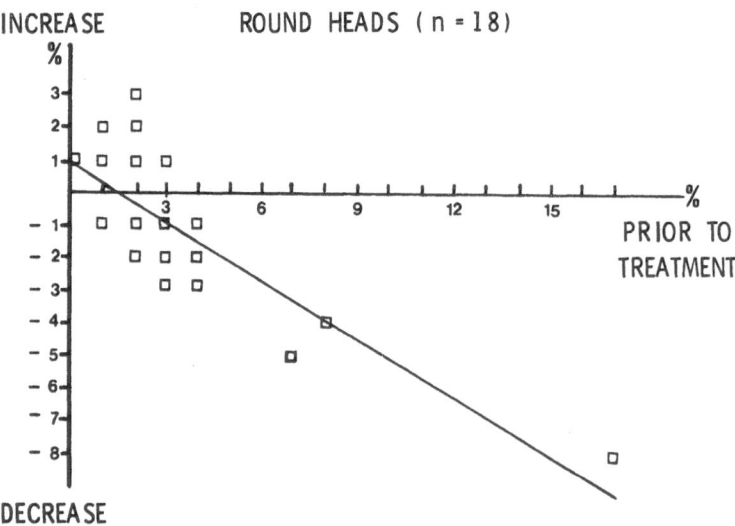

Figure 4 Effect of treatment with tamoxifen for 3 months (2×10 mg/day) on the percentage of round heads

29
Tamoxifen in the management of male subfertility – a retrospective analysis

G. LUNGLMAYR, U. MAIER and CH. KRATZIK

INTRODUCTION

Tamoxifen stimulates pituitary gonadotropin release by competing with oestrogens for the hypothalamic receptors[1-5]. It has a weaker intrinsic oestrogenic activity compared to clomiphene. Recently, attempts have been made to treat idiopathic oligozoospermia with tamoxifen, resulting in an increase of sperm count[6,7] as well as sperm motility[8] This paper has been designed to further elucidate the therapeutic effects of tamoxifen in idiopathic oligozoospermia.

PATIENTS AND METHODS

158 couples who had a history of infertility of 3–9 years were accepted into an open clinical trial. All males were normal on physical examination, and gave no history of inflammatory diseases of the genital tract, cryptorchidism or varicocele. Before treatment with tamoxifen a minimum of two ejaculates were investigated at an interval of 4–6 weeks. Semen samples were obtained by masturbation after a 5 day sexual abstinence. Semen analysis consisted of determination of the volume, pH, sperm count, motility and morphology. All individuals were found to be oligozoospermic, presenting with sperm between 8.1–17.6 million/ml and a total motility of sperms 14–48%. The investigation of sperm morphology resulted in a percentage of 23–41% of morphologically normal spermatozoa.

On 3 consecutive days, LH, FSH and testosterone were assayed in blood samples collected between 1500 h and 1700 h. The hormone concentrations were measured by radioimmunoassays. All methods have been previously described in detail[8]. Pretreatment levels of LH (3.1–8.3 mIU/ml), FSH (2.4–10.2 mIU/ml) and testosterone (3.2–6.8 ng/ml) were found to be within normal ranges as compared to normozoospermic age matched controls.

On routine gynaecological check-up no abnormalities indicating sub- or infertility of the females were reported. Hysterosalpingography and/or pertubation did not reveal any tubal factors. However, laparoscopies were not performed routinely so that minor adhesions could not be excluded.

Eighty-eight of the 158 patients accepted into this study had been unsuccessfully pretreated with various agents, including mesterolone, kallikrein and gonadotropins. They received no treatment for at least 6 months prior to the institution of tamoxifen therapy. 20 mg tamoxifen/day were administered for a period of 12 months. Treatment was discontinued earlier in 23 patients whose wives conceived under tamoxifen treatment within 1 year. Hormone levels and semen parameters were monitored at intervals of 3 months and statistically compared by the Wilcoxon test.

RESULTS

The endocrine profiles and semen parameters under tamoxifen are illustrated in the Figure 1. Tamoxifen produced a significant elevation of LH ($p < 0.05$),

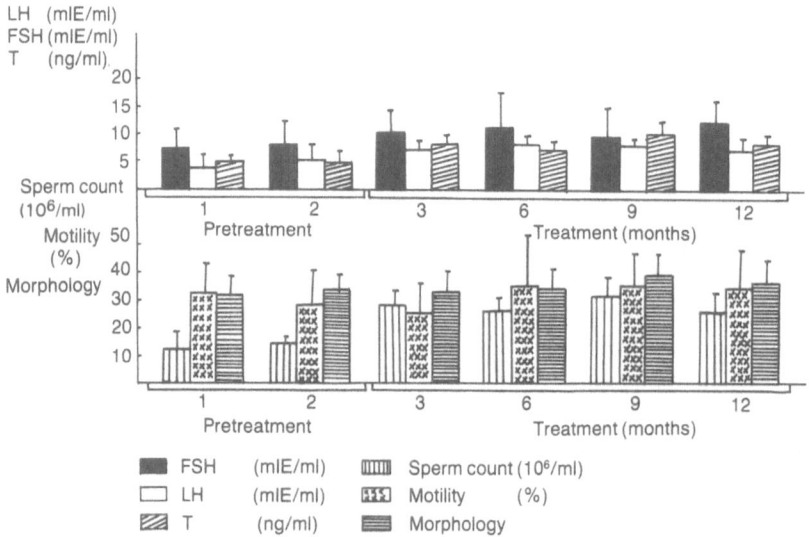

Figure 1 Endocrine profiles and semen parameters before and after treatment with tamoxifen (20 mg/day)

FSH ($p<0.001$) and testosterone ($p<0.001$). Daily intake of 20 mg of tamoxifen resulted in a sustained increase of the sperm count. Ejaculate volume, sperm motility as well as percentage of morphologically normal spermatozoa were not affected.

Twenty three couples became pregnant under tamoxifen treatment. Six conceptions occurred within 6 weeks in the remaining 17 between months 4 and 11 after the onset of treatment.

DISCUSSION

Patients presenting with moderate idiopathic oligozoospermia (sperm count > 5×10^6/ml) and normal gonadotropin plasma levels were selected for studying the effects of tamoxifen on endocrine profiles, semen parameters and conception rate. A significant elevation of LH, FSH and testosterone could be observed in all patients following the administration of the drug. The observation of a sustained increase of sperm count supports the assumption that spermatogenesis can be stimulated by tamoxifen in oligozoospermic males. However, the effect of tamoxifen on semen parameters seems to be confined to sperm count. There was no evidence of improvement of sperm motility and secretion of morphologically normal spermatozoa in this study.

The partners of 23 out of 158 oligozoospermic males conceived within 1 year under tamoxifen treatment. Six conceptions occurred within 6 weeks after the onset of therapy. They can hardly be related to a tamoxifen induced improvement of sperm quality, since the interval between institution of treatment and expected improvement of sperm count would be too short. The occurrence of those conceptions might rather be spontaneous and/or attributed to the psychological motivation of patients who have been accepted for a new promising treatment. The 17 males whose wives conceived between months 4 and 11 after the onset of tamoxifen therapy presented with a sperm count between $11–19 \times 10^6$/ml and a sperm motility between 31–42% 2 hours after delivery of the sample. In eight males out of 17 whose wives conceived under tamoxifen a relevant increase of sperm count was observed under treatment. It must be concluded from the results of this retrospective evaluation that the therapeutic effect of tamoxifen, in terms of increasing the conception rate of individuals presenting with idiopathic oligozoospermia, still remains questionable. A prospective controlled clinical trial seems to be necessary in order to clarify this problem.

SUMMARY

158 oligozoospermic males were treated with 20 mg of tamoxifen daily for 12 months. Tamoxifen produced a significant elevation in plasma levels of LH,

FSH and testosterone in all patients. A sustained increase of sperm count was observed under tamoxifen. Sperm motility and morphology were not affected. Twenty-three couples reported conception under treatment, occurring within the first 6 weeks in six cases and in 17 between months 4 and 11. A concomitant rise in sperm count was observed in 8 out of 17 individuals whose wives conceived. Evaluation of the therapeutic effect of tamoxifen necessitates further investigation in terms of prospective controlled clinical trials.

References

1. Commhaire, F. (1978). Hormonal effects of an antiestrogen, Tamoxifen, in normal and oligospermic men. *Fertil. Steril.*, **29**, 320
2. Lunan, C. B., Klopper, A. (1975). Antiestrogens, a review. *Clin. Endocrinol.*, **4**, 551
3. Patterson, J. S. (1981). Clinical aspects and development of antiestrogen therapy. A review of the endocrine effects of tamoxifen in animals and man. *J. Endocrinol.*, **89**, 67
4. Willis, K. J., London, D. R., Bevis, M. A., Butt, W. R., Lynch, S. S. and Holder, G. (1977). Hormonal effects of Tamoxifen in oligospermic men. *J. Endocrinol.*, **73**, 171
5. Comhaire, F. (1976). Treatment of Oligospermia with Tamoxifen. *Int. J. Fertil.*, **21**, 232
6. Schill, W. B., Landthaler, M. (1980). Tamoxifen treatment of Oligozoospermia. *Andrologia*, **12**, 546
7. Spona, J., Lunglmayr, G. (1974). Physiologie des hypophysär-testicularen Regulationssystems des Mannes; radioimmunologische Hormonuntersuchungen. *Wien. Klin. Wschr.*, **86**, 311
8. Bartsch, G., Scheiber, K. (1981). Tamoxifen Treatment in Oligozoospermia. *Eur. J. Urol.*, **7**, 283

30
Increased sperm count in 41 cases of idiopathic normogonadotropic oligozoospermia following treatment with tamoxifen

J. BUVAT, K. ARDAENS-BOULIER, A. LEMAIRE,
J. C. FOURLINNIE and M. BUVAT-HERBAUT

INTRODUCTION

Clomiphene citrate has often been used in the treatment of idiopathic oligozoospermia. This anti-oestrogenic drug increases serum gonadotropins and testosterone, which in turn may stimulate spermatogenesis. However, evidence is lacking that clomiphene citrate clearly improves semen quality in oligozoospermic males[1]. This poor effect on oligozoospermia has been attributed to the intrinsic oestrogenic activity of clomiphene citrate, hence a less oestrogenic drug may be more suitable for treating such males.

Tamoxifen also exhibits both anti-oestrogenic and oestrogenic effects. However, its oestrogenic effects seem weaker than those of clomiphene in human males[2]. Hence, we studied the effects of tamoxifen upon semen and hormones in 41 selected oligozoospermic males.

MATERIALS AND METHODS

Forty-one oligozoospermic males, 25–39 years old, were selected according to the following five criteria: (1) sperm concentration persistently less than 25×10^6 /ml (in most cases, reduced sperm motility was present), (2) no clear aetiology detected by interview or clinical examination, especially no history of orchitis, cryptorchidism, or varicocele, (3) basal serum FSH level in the normal range, (4) infertility dating back at least 2 years, (5) no major abnormality in the female partner capable of fully accounting for the infertility. Fertility was completely investigated in each female partner. Female fertility was absolutely normal in 13 cases. In the 28 other cases, minor abnormalities of ovulation, or of the preovulatory cervical mucus were found. These abnormalities were treated in conjunction with the administration of tamoxifen to the male partner.

The male patients were treated with 20 mg tamoxifen/day for 5–15 months. Two semen samples, obtained at a 3 month interval were analysed before treatment. At least two other semen samples, obtained at intervals of 2–3 months after the second month of treatment, were analysed during treatment. The mean values of the semen analyses performed before treatment were compared to the mean values of serum analyses performed during treatment with the paired t-test.

In 20 patients, an LHRH test (25 μg i.v.) was performed prior to the onset of treatment, in order to determine whether the gonadotropin response to LHRH was correlated to the subsequent sperm improvement. In addition, in 14 patients, serum FSH and LH, and plasma testosterone and oestradiol were determined before treatment, then after 2 and 12 weeks of treatment, the results were compared with paired t-test.

RESULTS

The mean values $\pm$ SE of semen characteristics before and during tamoxifen treatment are shown in Table 1. No significant change occurred with respect to semen volume, sperm motility, or sperm morphology. Conversely, a significant increase (two fold) of mean sperm concentration, and mean total

Table 1   Semen characteristics (mean $\pm$ SE) before treatment and during tamoxifen treatment (20 mg per day) in 41 oligozoospermic males

	Before treatment	During treatment	Statistical significance
Sperm volume (ml)	4.13±0.18	4.2±0.33	no
Sperm motility (% after 1 h)	50.6±2.9	51.3±3.2	no
Sperm morphology (% abnormal forms)	39.9±2	42.4±3.2	no
Sperm concentration ($\times 10^6$/ml)	11.94±1.12	23.62±3.67	$p<0.001$
Total sperm count/ ejaculate ($\times 10^6$)	65±5.95	113.32±27.43	$p<0.001$

sperm count per ejaculate was observed ($p<0.001$). A clear sperm improvement (during treatment sperm count at least ×2 and > 10 million/ml) occurred in 15 cases.

Fourteen pregnancies (34% of the 41 patients) were reported in the course of tamoxifen treatment (262 months in 25 patients). The pregnancy rates were about the same in the couples in which female fertility was absolutely normal (4 of the 13 patients, 30%) and in those in which female fertility was slightly disturbed (10 of the 28 patients, 35%). These pregnancies thus did not result from specific therapy given to the female partners.

The LHRH test was of no predictive value. The gonadotropin response to LHRH was exaggerated only in 3 of the 20 studied cases. Two pregnancies, associated with a clear sperm improvement, occurred in these three cases.

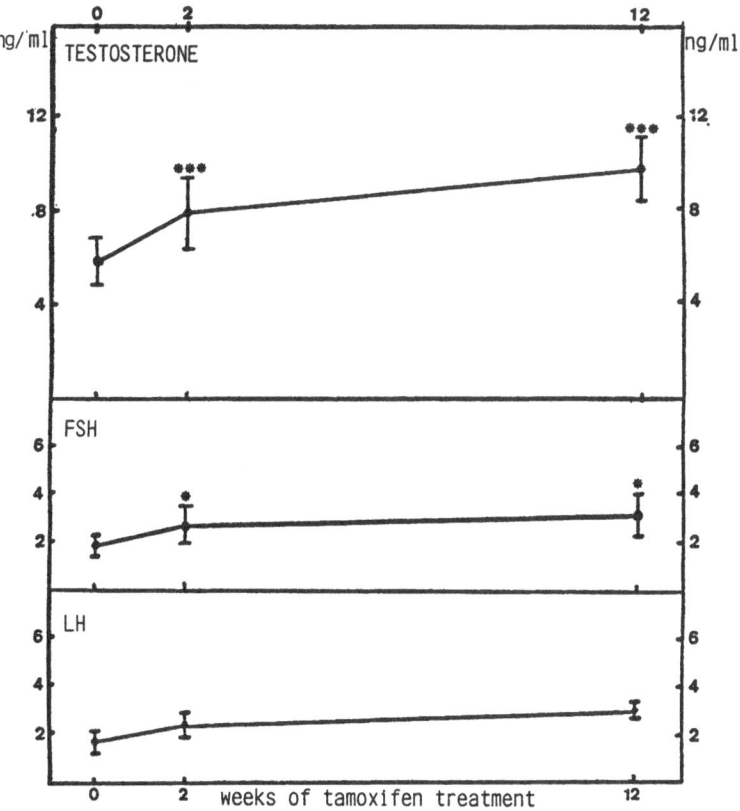

Figure 1   Plasma testosterone, serum LH and serum FSH levels (mean ± SE) in 14 oligozoospermic males before treatment, then after 2 weeks and 12 weeks of tamoxifen treatment (20 mg/day)
* ($p<0.05$ *** $p<0.001$ with respect to the pretreatment values

Serum LH and FSH, and plasma testosterone, increased during tamoxifen treatment, as shown in Figure 1. This increase was greater after 12 weeks than after 2 weeks of treatment, and was significant only for serum FSH ($p < 0.05$) and plasma testosterone ($p < 0.001$). Plasma oestradiol also increased during treatment (58 ± 10.7 vs 32.7 ± 4.2 pg/ml, $p < 0.01$), but the plasma testosterone/oestradiol ratio was not modified (164.2 ± 33.7 vs 158.7 ± 22.9).

DISCUSSION

Fertility improved in some of our 41 oligozoospermic males during longterm treatment with 20 mg tamoxifen per day. Similar results were reported by Vermeulen and Comhaire[2] in a group of comparable patients. However, a placebo effect of tamoxifen cannot be ruled out. A double blind vs placebo study would be necessary to confirm the tamoxifen induced improvement of fertility.

The effects of tamoxifen upon spermatogenesis may depend on the increased levels of gonadal hormones that this drug induces. Indeed FSH and testosterone are known to stimulate spermatogenesis, and our results confirm previous studies which showed that serum gonadotropins and plasma testosterone significantly increase during tamoxifen treatment in normal males as in oligozoospermic males[2]. In addition, a direct beneficial effect of tamoxifen upon spermatogenesis cannot be ruled out, since Δ1-testolactone, which decreases oestrogens without significantly changing the other gonadal hormones, increases sperm count in oligozoospermic males[3].

In conclusion, a regular intake of tamoxifen, 20 mg per day, improves fertility in certain oligozoospermic males, although a placebo effect cannot be ruled out. Thus tamoxifen may be advocated in cases of normogonadotropic oligozoospermia, since it is a convenient and relatively inexpensive treatment, with very few side effects.

ACKNOWLEDGEMENTS

We are indebted to Mrs Leserre for the preparation of the manuscript.

References

1. Newton, R., Schinfeld, J. S. and Schiff, I. (1980). Clomiphene treatment of infertile men: failure of response in idiopathic oligospermia. *Fertil. Steril.*, **34**, 399
2. Vermeulen, A. and Comhaire, F. (1978). Hormonal effects of an antiestrogen, tamoxifen, in normal and oligospermic men. *Fertil. Steril.*, **29**, 320
3. Vigersky, R. A. and Glass, A. R. (1981). Effects of Δ-1-testolactone on the pituitary testicular axis in oligospermic men. *J. Clin. Endocrinol. Metab.*, **52**, 897

31
Treatment of oligozoospermia with Chinese herb medicine (Hachimi-Jiou-Gan)

H. YOSHIDA, Y. NAITOH, M. WATANABE and K. IMAMURA

INTRODUCTION

In Japan, one of the Chinese herb medicines, Hachimi-jiou-gan (TJ-7), has been proved effective in reducing symptoms of prostatic hypertrophy and other prostatisms[1-3]. Since very few studies have been presented on its spermatogenic effect[4], we studied the clinical effect of this Chinese herb medicine for male infertility with oligozoospermia.

MATERIALS AND METHODS

Forty-nine patients with oligozoospermia, ranging in age from 24 to 42 years old, were treated by TJ-7, after giving their consent. Their wives had no gynaecological problems.

Table 1 Composition of Hachimi-jiou-gan, 'Paweidihuangwan' (Eight herb tonic tea, TJ-7) 5.0 g of this product contains 2.0 g of dried extract derived from mixed crude drugs as mentioned below

Jiou	: Rehmanniae Radix	6.0 g
San-shu-yu	: Corni Fructus	3.0 g
San-yaku	: Dioscoreae Rhizoma	3.0 g
Taku-sha	: Alisimatis Rhizoma	3.0 g
Buku-ryo	: Hoeien	3.0 g
Bo-tan-pi	: Moutan Cortex	2.5 g
Kei-hi	: Cinnamomi Cortex	1.0 g
Kakou-bu-shi	: Aconoti Tiber	0.5 g

(by Tsumura Juntendo, Inc. Tokyo, Japan)

In terms of sperm density, we categorized our patients into two groups: one was 'moderate oligozoospermia' (sperm density $10-40 \times 10^6$/ml), and the other was 'severe oligozoospermia' (sperm density below 10 million/ml).

We made comparisons of the best values of seminal analysis before and after TJ-7 therapy. We used the Student's paired t-test for statistical analysis.

TJ-7 is a preparation consisting of eight kinds of herbs as shown in Table 1. TJ-7 was administered orally at a dose of 2.5 g twice a day for more than 12 weeks. During TJ-7 therapy, we made it a rule to analyse their semen every 4 weeks.

RESULTS

Changes in sperm density and total sperm count in moderate oligozoospermia are shown in Figure 1. Many cases showed a marked increase in both seminal findings. The most remarkable point was that the change in sperm density and total sperm count occurred in a relatively short time, i.e. 4–8 weeks after starting the treatment.

Changes in the mean values of seminal analysis of 33 cases with moderate oligozoospermia are shown in Table 2. We observed a statistically significant improvement in ejaculate volume, sperm density, sperm motility, total sperm count and total count of motile spermatozoa. In 16 cases with severe oligozoospermia, we observed a statistically significant improvement except for volume and sperm density, as shown in Table 3.

The clinical effect of TJ-7 therapy is shown in Table 4. A marked improvement in sperm density was observed in 27 patients (55.1%). Among them, pregnancy occurred in the wives of 11 patients (22.5%).

Table 2 Changes in seminal analysis (means ± SD) (moderate oligozoospermia; sperm density, $10-40 \times 10^6$/ml)

$N=33$	Before	After	p^*
Volume (ml)	3.6±1.1	4.0±1.2	$p<0.05$
Sperm density (10^6/ml)	22.6±8.0	64.8±43.5	$p<0.01$
Sperm motility (%)	52.4±19.4	61.3±17.8	$p<0.01$
Total sperm count (10^6/semen)	83.3±45.9	251.1±179.2	$p<0.01$
Total count of motile spermatozoa (10^6/semen)	47.2±34.9	167.3±140.6	$p<0.01$

* paired t-test

156

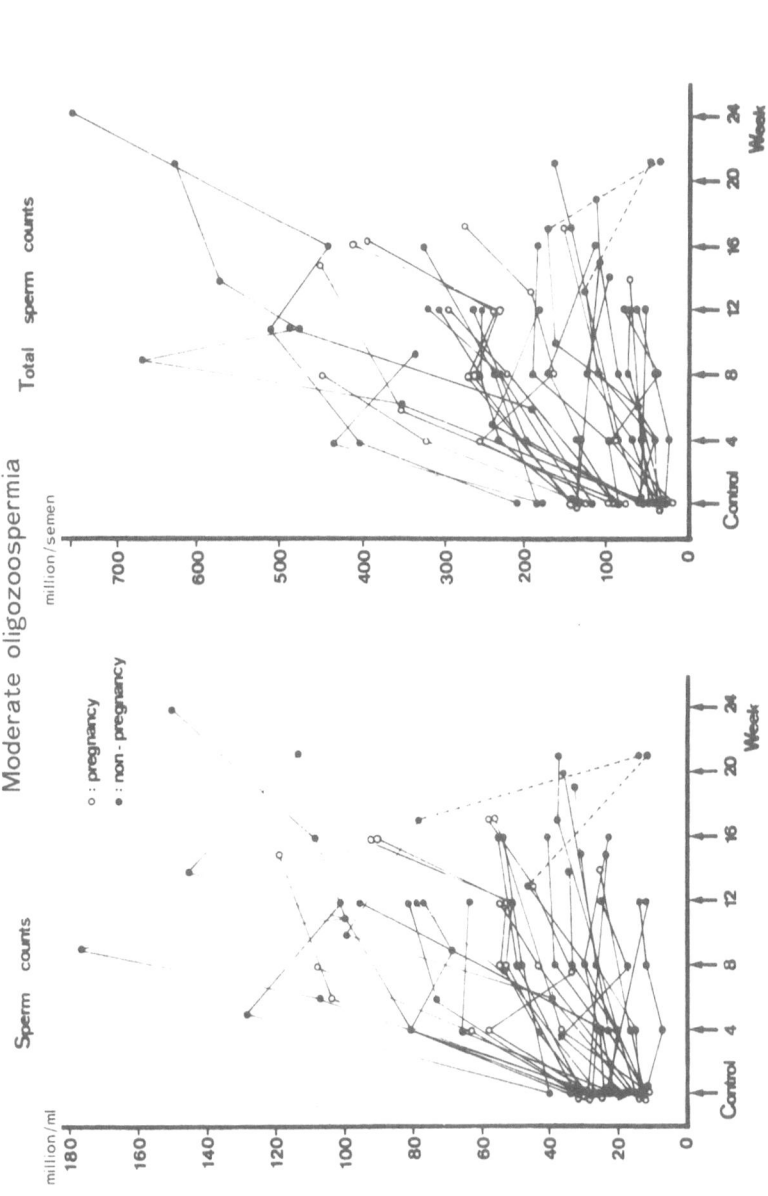

Figure 1 Changes in sperm count and total sperm count in cases of moderate oligozoospermia (Both findings in two patients fell after termination of TJ-7 administration (—))

Table 3   Changes in seminal analysis (means±SD) (severe oligozoospermia; sperm density, <10 million/ml)

$N=16$	Before	After	p^*
Volume (ml)	4.2±1.9	4.2±1.8	NS
Sperm density (10^6/ml)	3.8±3.2	18.8±32.0	NS
Sperm motility (%)	42.2±17.5	53.3±15.2	$p<0.01$
Total sperm count (10^6/semen)	17.2±19.7	82.2±155.7	$p<0.05$
Total count of motile spermatozoa (10^6/semen)	7.1±9.0	36.2±61.2	$p<0.05$

* paired t-test, NS: not significant

The criteria of clinical evaluation was as follows. *'Improvement'*: Sperm density improved to over 200%. In cases whose sperm density was below 5×10^6/ml, the clinical effect was evaluated when the sperm density improved to over 10×10^6/ml after treatment. *'Clinically effective cases'* included both pregnancy and improvement.

DISCUSSION

The pharmacological mechanism of TJ-7 action is not clear. Hsu and Peacher[5] have postulated, of the eight herbs composing TJ-7, that Jiou, San-shu-yu and San-yaku were used for alimentation and increasing sexual potency or libido, Buku-ryo and Taku-sha improve disorders of micturition, Bo-tan-pi relieves muscle tension or reduces anxiety, and Kakou-bu-shi increases regeneration.

Table 4   Evaluation of clinical effect

$N=49$	Moderate oligozoospermia	Severe oligozoospermia	Total
Cases	33	16	49
Pregnancy	9 (27.3%)	2 (12.5%)	11 (22.5%)
Improvement	11 (33.3%)	5 (31.3%)	16 (32.7%)
Clinical effect	20 (60.6%)	7 (43.8%)	27 (55.1%)

Although, Heller and Clermont[6] have established that it takes 74 days for a mature sperm to develop from a spermatogonium and the transport time of spermatozoa, from exit from the testis until storage in the distal cauda, is about 12 days in man[7], in our study many cases showed an improvement of sperm density as early as 4–8 weeks after treatment of TJ-7.

From these results, it is suggested that this Chinese herb medicine improved the blood circulation in testes and accessory organs and accelerated sperm transport.

Additionally, we consider that TJ-7 is more effective than other existing medicines as a treatment for oligozoospermia, and since it can be easily taken orally without any serious side effects, it will be a possible choice for primary treatment of idiopathic oligozoospermia, especially moderate oligozoospermia.

References

1. Niijima, T., Ueno, A. and Kawabe, K. (1979). Subjective relief from prostatism with a herb medicine. *Acta Urol. Jpn.*, **25**, 977
2. Arima, H., Sagawa, S. and Sonoda, T. (1979). Conservative therapy with hachimijiogan for micturition disturbances. *Acta Urol. Jpn.*, **25**, 1231
3. Kitagawa, R., Kano, S., Nishiura, H., Ogawa, Y. and Takahashi, S. (1980). Effects of hachimiohgan on bladder outlet obstruction. *Acta Urol. Jpn.*, **26**, 97
4. Yoshida, H. (1982). Male sterility – therapy of male sterility with Chinese herb medicine. *Sanfujinka-no-sekai*, **34**, 114
5. Hsu, H.-Y. and Peacher, W.G. (1976). *Chinese Herb Medicine and Therapy*, *Paweidihuangwan*, pp. 168–9. (Nashville, Tennessee: Oriental Healing Arts Institute Hawaiian Gardens, California and Aurora Publishers Incorporation)
6. Heller, C.G. and Clermont, Y. (1964). Kinetics of the germinal epithelium in man. *Recent Progr. Hormone Res.*, **20**, 545
7. Rowley, M.J., Teshima, F. and Heller, C.G. (1970). Duration of transit of spermatozoa through the human male ductular system. *Fertil. Steril.*, **21**, 390

32
Bacterial contamination of semen of infertile couples and the effect of antibiotic treatment of semen quality and fertility

M. SHILON, Y. STADTMAUER, M. HOLZINGER,
B. BARTOOV and C. BAHARY

ABSTRACT

A group of men under investigation for infertility has been studied with regard to findings of aerobic, anaerobic bacteria, ureaplasma and parameters of semen analysis indicating possible bacteriospermia. These parameters were: viscosity, sperm agglutination, high and low Ca^{2+} levels, Geimsa staining as well as possible prostatic message. The group comprised 110 men, 68 of which were diagnosed by one or more of the above parameters as having a possible genital tract infection. In 92% of the latter group teratozoospermia was demonstrated. Forty-six men out of this group were appropriately treated with antibiotics, among them 62.9% have shown a cyclic or steady improvement and the pregnancy rate was 39.1%. These results were significant ($p < 0.05$) when compared to the untreated group.

INTRODUCTION

In evaluating the infertile couple, the investigation and treatment of the male factor has become increasingly important as knowledge of this specific area has grown. While the investigation of female infertility spreads over many different fields using various tests, the investigation of male infertility concentrates mainly on semen analysis.

Several reports in recent literature deal with male genital tract infection and its possible negative influence on sperm quality, and accordingly on fertility. Yet a unified opinion among the investigators has as yet not been formulated[1-4].

In our work with infertile couples we attempted to examine the prevalence of various sperm infections among the males and the effect of treatment with different antibiotics.

MATERIALS AND METHODS

110 couples treated in our out-patient clinic underwent sperm analysis at our infertile research laboratory.

Semen was collected by means of masturbation, after careful washing of the penis especially the glans penis and urethral meatus with an antiseptic solution, into a sterile wide-mouthed jar. The patients were given clear instructions to preserve aseptic conditions. Semen analysis included, apart from routine parameters, special attention to the possible influence of infections on semen quality such as: culture for pathogenic micro-organisms or background bacteria over 3×10^3/ejaculate, viscosity sperm agglutination, calcium levels over 26 mg% or below 10 mg%, Geimsa staining of sperm for identification of bacteria, white blood cells and epithelial cells.

Aerobic and anaerobic cultures were made, as well as cultures for *Ureaplasma urealithium* and antibiograms. In all those cases where a possible bacterial contamination was suspected, the prostate was also examined, on average twice per patient. A routine rectal examination was performed, followed by a prostatic massage for emission of the secretion that was also cultured and examined cytologically. In all cases a urinary tract infection was excluded by means of urine analysis and cultures.

In those cases where a male genital tract infection was proven, suitable antibiotic treatment was administered for 2 weeks, after which semen prostate and bacterial cultures were re-examined.

In those cases where no improvement in semen analysis was noticeable and/or the cultures continued to be positive, a further antibiotic treatment for 6 weeks for both partners was prescribed, together with anticongestive drug treatment and multivitamins, all this under the repeated control of semen quality and hints of possible infection.

In most of the cases this treatment eradicated bacterial contamination, and only a few cases had to be treated for a further cycle.

RESULTS

Of the 110 men examined, 68 (62%) were suspected of semen contamination.

162

The distribution of the different parameters indicating possible bacterio-spermia among those patients is shown in Table 1. The diagnosis of possible bacteriospermia made on the basis of one parameter – 23 cases (34%), on the basis of two parameters – 26 cases (38%), on the basis of three parameters – 15 cases (22%) and on the basis of four parameters – 4 cases (6%). A list of the isolated bacteria and the distribution of their appearance among the patients examined is shown in Tables 2 and 3, respectively. Out of the 68 men with

Table 1 Distribution of parameters indicating possible bacteriospermia

Parameter	Number of cases	%
Bacterial growth	54	86
Viscosity	11	17
Sperm agglutination	12	19
Calcium, high or low	34	54
Prostatic massage	19	30
Geimsa staining, positive	18	26

Table 2 A list of bacteria isolated from semen cultures

Faecal bacteria:
1. *E. coli*
2. *Klebsiella* sp.
3. *Enterobacter* sp.
4. *Proteus* sp.
5. *Citrobacter* sp.
6. *Providencia* sp.

Normal skin flora:
1. *α-Streptococci*
2. *β-Streptococci*
3. *Staphylococcus albus*
4. *Diphteroides*
5. *Neisseria* sp.

Gram positive cocci:
1. *β-Haemolytic streptococcus* GR. A; GR. B
2. *Streptococcus faecalis*
3. *Staphylococcus aureus*

Anaerobic bacteria:
1. *Peptococci* sp.
2. *Peptostreptococci* sp.
3. *Bacteroides* sp.

Table 3 Distribution of isolated bacteria among patients

Bacteria	Number of cases	%
Faecal bacteria	10	18
Background bacteria	21	35
Anaerobic bacteria	3	6
Ureaplasma urealyticum	4	7
Faecal and background bacteria	5	9
Faecal bacteria and ureoplasma	1	2
Background bacteria and ureoplasma	2	4
Background and anaerobic bacteria	8	15
Total	54	100

Table 4 The effect of antibiotic treatment on semen analysis and pregnancy rate

Antibiotic treatment	Follow-up	No. cases	Abortion		Normal pregnancy		% preg.
No	No	16	1		1		
No	No improvement	4	1		0		
No	Cyclic improvement	2	0		0		
No	Total	22	2	+	1	=	13.6
Yes	No	19	2		5		
Yes	No improvement	10	3		0		
Yes	Cyclic improvement	8	0		3		
Yes	Steady improvement	9	0		5		
Yes	Total	46	5	+	13	=	39.1

suspected bacteriospermia only six (9%) were normozoospermia, with regards to semen analysis, the rest (92%) were defined as teratozoospermia, of which 36 cases (53%) were isolated teratozoospermia, six cases (9%) terato-astheno-zoospermia, five cases (7%) terato-oligozoospermia and 15 cases (22%) OTA. The percentage distribution of normal spermatozoa among these groups was 43 ± 5.6, 19.6 ± 8.9, 20 ± 13.6, 17.6 ± 8.5 and 12.7 ± 9.2, respectively.

Table 4 summarizes the effect of the antibiotic treatment on semen analysis and pregnancy rate. Out of 68 men suspected to have contaminated semen, 46 underwent antibiotic treatment, of which 27 had a thorough semen analysis follow-up in order to assess the efficiency of the treatment. Among them 10 cases (32.1%) showed no improvement in their semen analysis. In eight cases (29.6%) there was a cyclic improvement corresponding to the antibiotic treatment, and in nine cases (33.3%) a steady improvement in their semen was observed. In the treated groups 18 pregnancies (39.1%) were obtained, five of them spontaneously aborted (none from the improved semen analysis group) and 13 were normal pregnancies. Only three pregnancies (13.6%) were obtained in the untreated group, two of which aborted.

Although 60% of the follow-up treated patients showed improvement in semen quality, the rise in fertility was only 30%. That probably depended on an unexcluded female factor, nevertheless, semen quality as well as rate of pregnancy were significantly improved (p 0.05).

CONCLUSIONS

The high percentage of suspected bacteriospermia in men of infertile couples reported here is in agreement with the earlier publications of Dahlberg[5], Rehewy et al.[6] and Moberg et al.[3]. The high rate of teratozoospermia found among these men is in accordance with the report of McGowan et al.[7], which found that infection in the semen did not significantly affect the count, motility or volume of the specimen.

By means of massive antibiotic treatment it was possible to overcome the infections and markedly improve sperm quality and significantly elevate fertility.

In view of the results obtained it seems to us that there is ample justification to continue research in this field in the hope that, in this way, we may solve a significant problem in male infertility.

References

1. Eliasson, R. and Johannisson, E. (1978). Cytological studies of prostatic fluids from men with and without abnormal palpatory findings of the prostate. II. Clinical application. *Int. J. Androl.*, **1**, 582
2. Homonnai, T. Z., Sasson, S., Paz, G. and Kraicer, P. F. (1975). Improvement of fertility and semen quality in men treated with a combination of anticongestive and antibiotic drugs. *Int. J. Fertil.*, **20**, 45
3. Moberg, P. J., Emeroth, P., Ljung, A. and Nord, C. E. (1980). Bacterial flora in semen before and after Doxycycline treatment of infertile couples. *Int. J. Androl.*, **3**, 46
4. Toth, A. and Lesser, M. L. (1981). Asymptomatic bacteriospermia and infertile men. *Fertil. and Steril.*, **36**, 88
5. Dahlberg, B. (1976). Asymptomatic bacteriospermia. *Urology*, **8**, 563
6. Rehewy, M. S. E., Hafez, E. S. E., Thomas, A. and Brown, W. J. (1979). Aerobic and anaerobic bacterial flora in semen from fertile and infertile groups of men. *Arch. Androl.*, **2**, 263
7. McGowan, M. P., Burger, H. G., Baker, H. W., de Kretser, D. M. and Kovacs, G. (1981). The incidence of non-specific infection in the semen in fertile and sub-fertile males. *Int. J. Androl.*, **4**, 657

Section 5

Surgical Treatment
of the
Infertile Male

33
Effects on semen parameters and pregnancy rate after occlusion of the spermatic vein in subfertile men with idiopathic varicocele

U. MAIER, G. LUNGLMAYR, P. RIEDL and W. KUMPAN

INTRODUCTION

Since the exact pathogenetic mechanism by which a varicocele influences spermatogenesis has not yet been definitely clarified, the physical, thermal and hormonal noxae so far held responsible are still valid. Although all the theories about the connection between varicocele and subfertility can neither explain the simultaneous lesion of the contralateral testicle, which may be expressed in pathological parameters of the ejaculate, nor the frequently demonstrated fertility of individuals with varicoceles, the positive influence of spermatica ligature on male subfertility has been recognized since the publications by Tulloch[1], Braun[2], Dubin and Amelar[3].

After the many different procedures for surgical treatment of a varicocele (high ligature, ligation at the superficial or the deep inguinal ring, with or without simultaneous ligature of the accompanying artery, additional intra-operative phlebography in order to avoid a recurrent varicocele) selective transfemoral occlusion of the vena spermatica represents a new procedure, which – now technically fully developed – permits, after an overall observation period of 5 years, valid statements on the effectivity of this – non invasive – method.

MATERIAL AND METHODS

Obliteration of the vena spermatica was performed in 102 patients with idiopathic varicocele on the left side, during the years 1978–1983 at the Central Institute for Radiodiagnostics of the Vienna University. The occlusion was achieved – after transfemoral probing of the spermatic vein – by injection of 2–6 ml of a 3–4% solution of a hydroxypolyethoxydodecans (Aethoxysklerol) via a coaxial balloon catheter, following the technique described by Riedl[4]. The abdominal radiation dose of 100–150 mrad and the surface radiation dose of 50–100 mrad at the testicle, which are caused by the procedure, may be regarded as harmless for the germinal epithelium. All interventions were performed on out-patients. Successful occlusion was always verified by follow-up phlebography of the vena spermatica. The stop of the radiopaque medium after injection of the sclerosing agent can be clearly recognized (Figures 1 and 2).

The indication for sclerosation was in 65 cases an infertile marriage, 18 patients complained of pain, and in 14 cases the varicocele was discovered in the course of a general medical check-up. Five patients came to the andrological out-patient department of our hospital because of impaired erection.

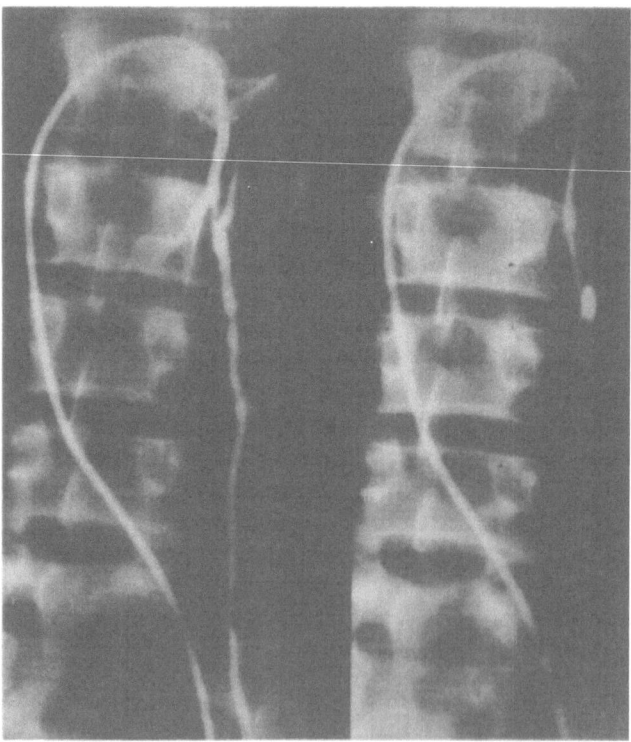

Figure 1 Phlebography of the spermatic vein before occlusion

Spermatological examinations before and after treatment were performed in 75 patients. The ejaculate was produced by masturbation after a period of sexual abstinence of at least 4 days. All spermiograms were evaluated by the same examiner. After registration of one or two pre-operative values, post-operative control spermiograms were taken – as far as possible – every 3–6 months for a period of up to 5 years, the best post-operative value being used for comparison. The pre-operative spermiograms of all patients were pathological according to Elliason's classification.

RESULTS

After occlusion no varicocele was demonstrable by clinical examination or plate thermography in 84% of the 75 patients who underwent spermatological control examinations; 10% showed a definite reduction of the venous convolution. This means a value of 6% real recurrences. Two of these five patients underwent successful surgical treatment by 'high ligation'. The

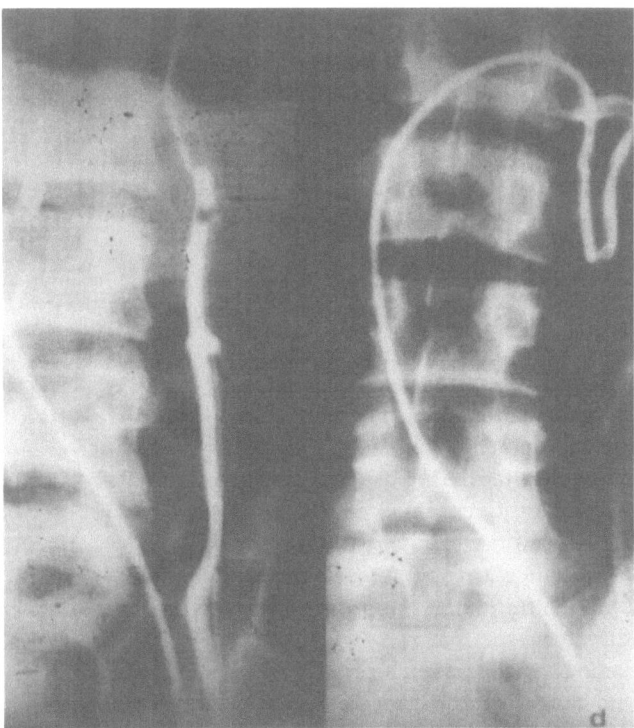

Figure 2 Phlebography of spermatic vein after occlusion

171

ejaculate was judged to be significantly improved, if at least one of the three spermatoparameters (sperm count, motility and normal forms) showed an increase of at least 50% of the initial value. Improvement of at least one of these parameters was registered in 72% of patients.

Sperm count was improved in 53.3% of the patients. The number of spermatozoa remained unchanged in almost one fourth of all patients (Table 1).

Spermatic motility showed an obvious increase in more than 50% of the patients, while deterioration of activity was registered in approximately 20% (Table 2).

Spermatic occlusion did not significantly influence spermatic morphology. Approximately the same number of cases showed either an increase or a decrease in the number of normal spermatozoa in the differential spermiogram (Table 3).

Twenty-one women out of 65 marriages (32.3%), which had remained infertile until the time of the operation, became pregnant within 6–32 months after treatment of their husbands. The birth of 24 healthy children by 20 women was registered. One woman had two miscarriages (Table 4).

Retrospective analysis of the spermiograms of those patients who were able to induce pregnancy after the operation – pre- and post-operative spermiograms were evaluated in 45 of 65 patients – furnished the same information about alterations of the spermiogram as that of the total population of the study. Normozoospermia – according to Elliason – was achieved in only two cases. It is striking that gravidity also occurred in the case of a patient whose spermiogram never showed more than 7×10^6 spermatozoa/ml and a motility of 13%.

DISCUSSION

Although relapses after transfemoral sclerosation of the spermatic vein are more frequent than after surgical ligature (Klosterhalfen[5] reports a 1% relapse rate after more than 500 high ligations), this non-invasive procedure of sclerosation, which hardly imposes any strain on the patient, appears to be a true alternative to surgical intervention, since the effect on spermatogenesis demonstrated by improved quality of the ejaculate[2,3,6,7] in about 70% is almost identical. Also a pregnancy rate of more than 30% in subfertile males compares well with the figures quoted in the literature for pregnancies after ligation of the vena spermatica.

When comparing the patients of the present study with 44 patients in our hospital who had undergone high ligation of the vena spermatica (ligature and sclerosation were placed approximately at the same local point in the spermatic vein), we found the changes in the parameters of the ejaculate to be

Table 1 Changes in sperm count after occlusion of spermatic vein ($n = 75$)

Density ↑	53.3%
No changes	24.0%
Density ↓	22.6%

Table 2 Changes in sperm-motility after occlusion of spermatic vein ($n = 75$)

Motility ↑	50.6%
No changes	29.4%
Motility ↓	20.0%

Table 3 Changes in sperm-morphology after occlusion of spermatic vein ($n = 75$)

Normal forms ↑	30.6%
No changes	36.1%
Normal forms ↓	33.3%

Table 4 Pregnancy rate after occlusion of spermatic vein in infertile marriage ($n = 65$)

21/65 = 32.3%	
24	Deliveries of healthy children
2	Abortions

very similar, however the rate of pregnancies after occlusion was almost twice as high[8].

On the basis of the data presented occlusion of the vena spermatica may definitely be recommended as a first step in the treatment of idiopathic varicocele.

References

1. Tulloch, W. S. (1955). Varicocele in subfertility: results of treatment. *Br. Med. J.*, **2**, 356
2. Brown, J. S. (1976). Varicocelectomy in the subfertile male: a ten year experience with 295 cases. *Fertil. Steril.*, **27**, 1046
3. Dubin, L. and Amelar, R. D. (1975). Varicocelectomy as therapy in male infertility: a study of 504 cases. *Fertil. Steril.*, **26**, 217
4. Riedl, P. (1979). Selektive Phlebographie und Katheterthrombosierung der Vena testicularis bei primärer Varikocele. *Wien. Klin. Wochenschr.*, **91** (Suppl.), 99

5. Klosterhalfen, H., Schirren, C. and Wagenknecht, L. V. (1979). Pathogenese und Therapie der Varikocele. *Urol. A.*, **18**, 187
6. Newton, R., Schinfeld, J. S. and Schiff, I. (1980). The effect of varicocelectomy on sperm count, motility and conception rate. *Fertil. Steril.*, **34**, 250
7. Maier, U. and Lunglmayr, G. (1982). Spermatologische Veränderungen nach Ligatur der Vena spermatica bei idiopathischer Varikozele. *Wien. Klin. Wochenschr.*, **94**, 240
8. Maier, U., Lunglmayr, G. and Riedl, P. (1982). Spermatologische Veränderungen nach Sklerosierung bzw. Ligatur der Vena spermatica bei idiopathischer Varikozele. *Akt. Urol.*, **13**, 300

34
Varicocelectomy for oligozoospermia

N. ANANDAN, R. C. L. FENELEY and J. C. GINGELL

SUMMARY

Eighty-four oligozoospermic patients with varicocele were treated by varicocelectomy. Improvement in the sperm count was noted in 71 patients (84.5%),
motility in 63 patients (75%) and pregnancy was achieved in 38 (45.2%).
Varicocelectomy also improved the sperm morphology and this was a
favourable factor in achieving pregnancy. Abnormalities of FSH, LH and
testosterone were noted in 15 patients (17%) and the significance is discussed.

INTRODUCTION

The success rate of varicocelectomy in terms of improvement of sperm
density, motility and morphology varies considerably in the many reported
series[1-3]. At present, there are no clear guidelines that enable the clinician to
anticipate which patient will benefit from the operation. We report the results
of our own series of patients operated upon between 1974–1981, and examine
the various factors influencing the outcome of surgery.

PATIENTS

A study of the case notes of 100 patients who underwent varicocelectomy for
oligozoospermia between 1974–1981 has been undertaken. Twelve patients
have been excluded in whom adequate detailed pre- or post-operative semen
analyses could not be retrieved. Four further patients have been excluded as in
three cases their wives were subsequently demonstrated to have bilateral
fallopian tube occlusion, and one patient had a high titre of antisperm

antibodies. This study is based upon the remaining 84 patients. The patients were aged between 27–48 years (mean 33.1 years). All of the patients had at least two semen analyses before operation, and after surgery further semen analyses were undertaken commencing 3–6 months post-operatively.

In all patients the varicocelectomy was undertaken via the inguinal canal, and any dilated veins of the cremasteric complex were also ligated. Six patients underwent bilateral varicocelectomy. Five patients had a recurrent varicocele, one of whom underwent further surgery; three patients developed left hydrocoele, two of whom required surgery.

RESULTS

Semen analysis

Sperm density

An increase in sperm count was achieved in 71 patients after operation, and those patients who made their wives pregnant had a better sperm count than those who did not (Tables 1 and 2).

Motility

An improvement in the percentage of motile sperms was noted in the ejaculate of 63 of the patients after varicocelectomy. The percentage of motile sperms

Table 1 Relation between post-operative sperm density and pregnancy rate

Patient group	No. of cases	Pregnancy No.	%
Post-operative increase in sperm density	71	35	49.2
No change in post-operative sperm density	13	3	23.0

Table 2 Pre-operative and post-operative sperm density and motility in patients who achieved pregnancy and those who did not

Patient group	Mean pre-operative sperm density $(10^6/ml)$	Motility (%)	Mean post-operative sperm density $(10^6/ml)$	Motility (%)
Pregnancy	19.3	33.8	54.9	49
No pregnancy	16.7	29.0	37.1	44.5

was greater in those patients who achieved pregnancy as compared with those that did not (Table 2).

Morphology

There was an increased number of morphologically abnormal sperms, mainly tapered heads, in the pre-operative ejaculate of 32 patients. After varicocelectomy, morphology returned to normal in 11 patients and 8 of whom made their wives pregnant. Successively fewer pregnancies were achieved with an increasing percentage of persisting morphologically abnormal forms (Table 3).

Hormone studies

Seven patients were noted to have an elevated FSH level and two patients had a raised LH level. Both FSH and LH levels were raised in four patients and the serum testosterone was low in two patients. The influence of varicocelectomy

Table 3 Relationship between abnormal sperm morphology and pregnancy

% Abnormality	Number of cases		Number of pregnancies
	Pre-op	Post-op	
up to 25%	3	2	1
26–50%	12	8	3
51–75%	13	6	1
> 76%	4	5	0
Normal	0	11	8
Total	32	32	13

Table 4 Results of variococelectomy in patients with elevated FSH

Patient no.	FSH (IU/l)	Pre-operative sperm density (10^6/ml)	Motility (%)	Post-operative sperm density (10^6/ml)	Motility (%)	Pregnancy
1	20	4	25	25	60	+
2	25	70	5	154	20	+
3	24	5	60	3	66	+
4	9.7	25	20	22	30	−
5	24	1.5	—	< 1	—	−
6	8.2	48	25	55	30	−
7	9.4	8	35	17	40	−

Table 5 Results of variococelectomy in patients with elevated LH

Patient no.	LH (IU/l)	Mean pre-operative sperm density (10⁶/ml)	Motility (%)	Mean post-operative sperm density (10⁶/ml)	Motility (%)	Pregnancy
1	11.1	30	25	107	70	+
2	13.5	6	40	25	30	+

Table 6 Results of variococelectomy in patients with elevated FSH and LH

Patient no.	FSH (IU/l)	LH (IU/l)	Pre-operative sperm density (10⁶/ml)	Motility (%)	Post-operative sperm density (10⁶/ml)	Motility (%)	Pregnancy
1	11.3	10.7	9	2	35	30	—
2	44	24	<1	10	2	90	—
3	25	15	2	20	30	50	-
4	23	12.2	8	50	12	80	—

Table 7 Results of variococelectomy in patients with low testosterone levels

Patient no.	Testosterone (IU/l)	Mean pre-operative sperm density (10⁶/ml)	Motility (%)	Mean post-operative sperm density (10⁶/ml)	Motility (%)	Preganancy
1	2.9	1	10	2	20	—
2	5.8	48	25	55	30	—

on semen analysis and the achievement of pregnancy in these patients is shown (Tables 4–7).

DISCUSSION

In our series an encouraging improvement in sperm density, motility and morphology was observed in many patients following varicocelectomy. The pregnancy rate in those patients in whom such an improvement occurred was approximately double that observed where there was no improvement in sperm quality. Apart from the few patients with both elevated LH and FSH levels and clinically small testes in whom the results of varicocelectomy were poor, no other predictive indices were detected. In particular the size of the varicocele and the size and consistency of the left testicle had no bearing on the outcome of surgery in respect of the semen quality.

Further studies are needed to establish why some oligozoospermic patients benefit from varicocelectomy while others are uninfluenced by surgery.

References

1. Dubin, L. and Amelar, R. D. (1975). Varicocelectomy as therapy in male infertility: A study of 504 cases. *Fertil. Steril.*, **26**, 217
2. Brown, J. S. (1976). Varicocelectomy in sub-fertile male. A ten year experience with 295 cases. *Fertil. Steril.*, **27**, 1046
3. Newton, R., Schifeld, J. S. and Schiff, I. (1980). The effect of varicocelectomy on sperm count, motility and conception rate. *Fertil. Steril.*, **34**, 250

35
Emission failure due to retroperitoneal lymphadenectomy: first report of a pregnancy after insemination of spermatozoa obtained by midodrin-induced retrograde ejaculation

W.-B. SCHILL and W. BOLLMANN

Retroperitoneal lymphadenectomy performed in patients with non-semi-nomatous testicular tumours causes, in most cases, ejaculatory impotence with aspermia owing to either retrograde ejaculation or to failure of emission. The type of ejaculatory impotence depends on the extensiveness of lymph-adenectomy. On the other hand, patients are usually potent and experience normal orgasm after these extensive operations.

The inability to produce an ejaculate is due to sympathetic denervation of the bladder neck, the vas deferens, the epididymis and the accessory sex glands leading to infertility[1]. Denervation does not allow contractions of the smooth muscles stimulating propulsion of spermatozoa and emission of the secretions of the accessory sex glands into the posterior urethra.

The diagnosis of ejaculatory failure is given by the patient's history of dry orgasm and the finding of aspermia. Differentiation between emission failure, also called transport aspermia, and retrograde ejaculation is possible by looking at the post-ejaculatory urine: in the case of transport aspermia the urine is clear and spermatozoa are missing in the sediment. The fructose test is negative. In the case of retrograde ejaculation, the post-ejaculatory urine specimen is opalescent, contains considerable amounts of spermatozoa and shows a positive fructose test.

For the treatment of aspermia the following possibilities have to be considered:

(1) Induction of antegrade or retrograde ejaculation by α-sympatho-mimetic or anticholinergic drugs,
(2) Recovery of spermatozoa from post-ejaculatory urine specimens and insemination, and
(3) Reconstructive surgery of the bladder neck or collection of epididymal spermatozoa by an alloplastic spermatocele.

Since the vas deferens, the seminal vesicles and the bladder neck closure are under adrenergic control, via adrenergic receptors, and are relaxed by para-sympathetic fibres via cholinergic receptors, the aim of pharmacological therapy is to increase sympathetic or to decrease parasympathetic tension leading to a relative increase of the sympathetic stimulation.

The following drugs were successfully used to induce antegrade ejaculation in men with retrograde ejaculation:

α-Sympathomimetic drugs
Phenylpropanolamine (Ornade) 2 × 1 capsule/day
Oxedrine (Synephrine) 60 mg i.v.
Midodrin (Gutron) 5–15 mg i.v. or 3 × 5 mg, oral
Imipramine (Tofranil) 25–75 mg/day, oral

Anticholinergic drugs
Brompheniramine (Dimothane, Ebalin) 2 × 8 mg/day, oral

However, to date, no pregnancies have been obtained by normal coitus during drug-induced antegrade ejaculation in patients with retrograde ejaculation. All known pregnancies, summarized in Table 1, were achieved by instrumental insemination of spermatozoa recovered without drugs in different ways from the bladder after retrograde ejaculation. Only two pregnancies were reported after instrumental insemination of semen obtained during pharmacological correction of a retrograde ejaculation into an antegrade ejaculation, by using the α-sympathomimetic drug phenylpropano-lamine (Ornade)[2]. On the other hand, pregnancies have never been obtained in cases of emission failure (transport aspermia). Thus, the result of treatment in men with anejaculation is rather moderate concerning achievement of pregnancy, and require an excellent cooperation between andrologists and gynaecologists. We report here the first successful case of a pregnancy in a patient with emission failure.

The patient is a 32 year old physician, who has been married for 5 years. The couple already have one child. In September 1979 the patient had to undergo orchiectomy and retroperitoneal lymph node dissection for a teratocarcinoma

182

Table 1 Conceptions achieved after insemination of spermatozoa recovered from the urine of men with retrograde ejaculation

Author	Number of conceptions
Fischer and Coats[4]	1
Hotchkiss et al.[5]	3
Walters and Kaufman[6]	1
Spira[7]	1
Rieser[8]	1
Günther[9]	1
Anselmo[10]	1
Bourne et al.[11]	1
Roo[12]	1
Bol[13]	1
Fuselier et al.[14]	1
Glezerman et al.[15]	2
Schram[16]	1
Sina[17]	1
Marmar et al.[18]	3
Crich and Jequier[19]	2
Kapetanakis et al.[20]	1
Kragt and Schellen[21]	1
Barwin et at[22]	7
Mahadevan et al.[23]	1
Colpi et al.[24]	1
Total number of conceptions	33

of the left testis. Since tumour stage I was found, no post-operative treatment was necessary. After surgery anejaculation was noticed, and a transport aspermia was diagnosed due to exclusion of retrograde ejaculation by sperm-free post-masturbatory urine specimens.

To induce semen emission and ejaculation, an intravenous bolus injection of 15 mg of the α-andrenergic receptor stimulating drug midodrin[3] (Gutron) was found suitable to achieve repeatedly retrograde ejaculation. Post-ejaculatory urine specimens showed between $26-330 \times 10^6$ spermatozoa of normal morphology. Total motility was 1-2%, progressive motility 1%. Alkalization of the urine by pentacitrate did not improve sperm motility. However, when the voided bladder was filled with 50 ml of Tyrode's solution, sperm motility improved up to 20% with 5% progressively motile spermatozoa. Addition of 4% bovine serum albumin to the sperm suspension showed no further improvement in motility. The following procedure for semen collection was found useful for the purpose of insemination:

(1) Voiding of the bladder,
(2) Sterile catheterization of the bladder using local anaesthesia (Instillagel),

(3) Instillation of 50 ml Tyrode's solution,
(4) Removal of catheter,
(5) Intravenous injection of 15 mg midodrin (3 ampoules Gutron),
(6) Masturbation followed by urination immediately and after 10 min,
(7) Centrifugation of urine specimen (10 min, 1000 r.p.m.),
(8) Resuspension of the sperm pellet in 1.5 ml Tyrode's solution and
(9) Insemination (0.5 ml intracervical, 1 ml precervical using a cervical adapter).

The 28 year old wife, who had delivered a healthy boy in 1978, had regular ovulatory cycles with ovulations around the 14th to 20th cycle day. During the first insemination cycle on day 16 the right ovary showed a ripe follicle of 18 mm diameter visualized by ultrasonography. The Insler score was 10. After retrieval of semen from the bladder 39×10^6 spermatozoa were inseminated, which showed a good forward motility with a mean velocity of $47 \mu m/s$. 36 hours later completed ovulation could be confirmed by ultrasonography on cycle day 18, thus making further inseminations unnecessary. A post-coital test performed at that time still showed 3–5 spermatozoa/HPF with good motility. Nine days after insemination conception could be diagnosed by an early morning urine hCG measurement. Spontaneous delivery of a healthy girl occurred at term. Serological investigations of different blood group antigens and of subgroups of the HLA system confirmed paternity.

In conclusion, induction of emission in patients with transport aspermia is possible using sympathomimetic agents, leading either to antegrade or retrograde ejaculation. In the case of a drug-induced retrograde ejaculation, retrieval of semen from the bladder and instrumental insemination is necessary to achieve a pregnancy. However, successful treatment depends mainly on close andrological–gynaecological co-operation.

ACKNOWLEDGEMENT

Determination of different blood group antigens and subgroups of the HLA system in the father, mother and child was kindly performed by Prof. Dr W. Mempel, Transfusionszentrum, Klinikum Großhadern, University of Munich.

References

1. Narayan, P., Lange, P. H. and Fraley, E. E. (1982). Ejaculation and fertility after extended retroperitoneal lymph node dissection for testicular cancer. *J. Urol.*, **127**, 685
2. Thiagarajah, S., Vaughan, E. D. and Kitchin, J. D. (1978). Retrograde ejaculation: successful pregnancy following combined sympathomimetic medication and insemination. *Fertil. Steril.*, **30**, 96
3. Jonas, D., Linzbach, P. and Weber, W. (1979). The use of midodrin in the treatment of ejaculation disorders following retroperitoneal lymphadenectomy. *Eur. Urol.*, **5**, 184

4. Fischer, J. C. and Coats, E. C. (1954). Sterility due to retrograde ejaculation of semen. *Obstet. Gynecol.*, **4**, 352
5. Hotchkiss, R. S., Pinto, A. B. and Kleegman, S. (1955). Artificial insemination with semen recovered from the bladder. *Fertil. Steril.*, **6**, 37
6. Walters, D. and Kaufman, M. S. (1959). Sterility due to retrograde ejaculation of semen. *Am. J. Obstet. Gynecol.*, **78**, 274
7. Spira, R. (1960). Artificial insemination after intrathecal injection of neostigmine in a paraplegic. *Lancet*, **1**, 670
8. Rieser, C. (1961). The etiology of retrograde ejaculation and a method for insemination. *Fertil. Steril.*, **12**, 488
9. Günther, E. (1967). Beitrag zur Kenntnis des Aspermatismus. *Derm. Wschr.*, **153**, 849
10. Anselmo, J. (1971). Successful homologous artificial insemination in a case of retrograde ejaculation. *Rev. Child. Obstet. Gynecol.*, **36**, 293
11. Bourne, R. B., Kretzschmar, W. A. and Esser, J. H. (1971). Successful artificial insemination in a diabetic with retrograde ejaculation. *Fertil. Steril.*, **22**, 275
12. Roo, H. (1972). Succesvolle inseminatie met post coitum urine bij retrospermie (cited in Colpi *et al.*[24])
13. Bol, J. J. (1973). Successful artificial insemination with spermatozoa recovered from the urine in a case of retrograde ejaculation. *Eur. J. Obstet. Gynecol. Reprod. Biol.*, **3**, 89
14. Fuselier, H. A., Schneider, G. T. and Ochsner, M. G. (1976). Successful artificial insemination following retrograde ejaculation. *Fertil. Steril.*, **27**, 1214
15. Glezerman, M., Lunenfeld, B., Potashnik, G., Oelsner, G. and Beer, R. (1976). Retrograde ejaculation: pathophysiologic aspects and report of two successfully treated cases. *Fertil. Steril.*, **27**, 796
16. Schram, J. (1976). Retrograde ejaculation: a new approach to therapy. *Fertil. Steril.*, **27**, 1216
17. Sina, D. (1976). Konzeptionsmöglichkeit bei der retrograden Ejakulation. In Kaden, R., Lübke, F. and Schirren, C. (eds.) *Fortschritte der Fertilitätsforschung III*, pp. 153–6. (Berlin: Grosse Verlag)
18. Marmar, J., Praiss, D. and De Benedictis, T. (1977). Post-coital voiding insemination technique for patients with retrograde ejaculation and infertility. *Urology*, **9**, 288
19. Crich, J. P. and Jequier, A. M. (1978). Infertility in men with retrograde ejaculation: the action of urine on sperm motility and a simple method for achieving antegrade ejaculation. *Fertil. Steril.*, **30**, 572
20. Kapetanakis, E., Rao, R., Dmowski, W. P. and Scommegna, A. (1978). Conception following insemination with a freeze-pressered retrograde ejaculate. *Fertil. Steril.*, **29**, 360
21. Kragt, F. and Schellen, A. (1978). Clinical report about some cases with retrograde ejaculation. *Andrologia*, **10**, 381
22. Barwin, B. N., McKay, D., Jolly, E. E. and Dempsey, A. (1980). Retrograde ejaculation. In Emperaire, J. C., Audebert, A. and Hafez, E. S. E. (eds.) *Homologous Artificial Insemination*, pp. 127–37. (The Hague: Martinus Nijhoff)
23. Mahadevan, M., Leeton, J. F. and Trounson, A. D. (1981). Noninvasive method of semen collection for successful artificial insemination in a case of retrograde ejaculation. *Fertil. Steril.*, **36**, 243
24. Colpi, G. M., Sommadossi, L. and Zanollo, A. (1983). Infertility caused by retrograde ejaculation: a successfuly treated case. *Andrologia*, **15**, 592

36
Restoration of antegrade ejaculation following radical retroperitoneal lymphadenectomy

D. KRÖPFL, M. MEYER-SCHWICKERATH, G. PLEWA,
R.-H. RINGERT and R. HARTUNG

INTRODUCTION

Retroperitoneal lymphadenectomy in patients with testicular cancer is followed by ejaculation disorders[1] in more than 80%. Since multimodal treatment has greatly improved the survival rate, side-effects such as infertility become more important, especially in the age group seen in men with cancer of the testis.

PATIENTS AND METHODS

Forty-three patients with ejaculation disorders after retroperitoneal lymphadenectomy underwent an andrological examination. Twenty-three showed loss of seminal emission, 18 had retrograde ejaculation and two a partial retrograde ejaculation. The mean age of these patients was 29 years.

Treatment with imipramine 25 mg given orally three times a day was initiated. After restoration of antegrade ejaculation, the dosage was reduced to 25 mg imipramine daily. Eleven patients were lost to follow-up, 32 underwent a repeated andrological examination.

RESULTS

Thirty-two out of 43 patients are still controlled. Six out of 17 presenting with loss of seminal emission initially regained antegrade ejaculation. Twelve out of 13 men showing retrograde ejaculation and both men with partial retrograde ejaculation regained antegrade ejaculation, too. In total, ejaculation was restored in 62.5% of patients (Table 1).

Table 1

	Controlled n	Antegrade ejaculation n (%)
Loss of seminal emission	17	6 (35)
Retrograde ejaculation	13	12 (92)
Partial retrograde ejaculation	2	2 (100)
Total	32	20 (62.5)

The volume of ejaculated spermatic fluid ranged from 3.2 to 0.9 ml. Four men showed normozoospermia, 13 patients showed oligozoospermia and two patients teratozoospermia. One shows asthenozoospermia. One patient fathered a daughter. In most patients restoration of antegrade ejaculation was achieved 48 h after the first medication. The maintenance dose was 25 mg imipramine daily (Table 2).

Table 2 Imipramine treatment

	Antegrade ejaculation observed	
	n	after
3×25 mg imipramine	28	1 day
	1	2 days
	1	10 days
	1	2 months
	1	6 months

Maintenance dose: 25 mg/day, $n = 12$

Side-effects were frequently seen. Dry mouth, blurred vision and sleep disturbances were the most prominent disorders.

DISCUSSION

Imipramine is a tricyclic antidepressant with a potent sympathomimetic effect[2]. The extensive α-adrenergic innervation of the epididymis, vas deferens, prostate gland and bladder neck muscle[3] explains the efficacy of imipramine in treating ejaculation disorders[4-7].

The presented results, obtained in a comparatively large group of patients, are very promising. Imipramine is an effective drug with which to treat patients presenting with a loss of seminal emission and/or retrograde ejaculation after lymphadenectomy. Side-effects are seen in most patients.

References

1. Albrecht, D. and Nagel, R. (1972). Verlust der Potentia generandi nach RLA bei malignen Hodentumoren. *Akt. Urol.*, 4, 91
2. Goodman, L. S. and Gilman, A. (eds.) (1965). *The Pharmacological Basis of Therapeutics*, pp. 198–204. (Saint Louis: Macmillan)
3. Sjöstrand, N. O. (1965). The adrenergic innervation of the vas deferens and the accessory male genital glands. *Acta Physiol. Scand.*, 65 (Suppl. 257), 1–82
4. Brooks, M. E., Berezin, M. and Braf, Z. (1980). Treatment of retrograde ejaculation with imipramine. *Urology*, 15, 353
5. Jonas, D., Linzbach, P. and Weber, W. (1977). Behandlung der retrograden Ejakulation nach retroperitonealer Lymphadenektomie mit Midodrin. *Urologe B*, 17, 49
6. Kelly, M. E. and Needle, M. A. (1979). Imipramine for aspermia after lymphadenectomy. *Urology*, 13, 414
7. Stockamp, K., Schreiter, F. and Altwein, J. E. (1974). Alpha-adrenergic drugs in retrograde ejaculation. *Fertil. Steril.*, 25, 817

37
Transurethral resection of verumontanum for ejaculatory duct stenosis and oligozoospermia

C. C. CARSON

ABSTRACT

While it's well known that trauma and infection cause ejaculatory duct stenosis, the use of vasography for the diagnosis and treatment planning of men with profound oligozoospermia is controversial. We evaluated 27 selected men for hypofertility with azoospermia using vasography. Four of these men had an obstruction identified in the distal ejaculatory duct at the level of the verumontanum on vasography. A history of gonococcal urethritis was obtained in two patients, urethral trauma in one patient, while the remaining patient had no significant genitourinary history except mild prostatitis. Testicular biopsies and gonadotropin studies were normal in all cases. Transurethral resection of the verumontanum was carried out in all cases, allowing efflux of contrast material on vasography. Sperm counts returned to a fertile range in one patient and markedly improved to oligozoospermic levels in two remaining patients. One patient remained azoospermic after surgery, despite an increased ejaculatory volume and return of fructose to his ejaculate.

Vasography is an important study in patients with profound oligozoospermia, especially if a history of gonococcal urethritis or urethral trauma can be elicited. Transurethral resection of the verumontanum is effective treatment for those patients with documented distal ejaculatory obstruction as a cause of their infertility.

Infertility caused by bilateral ejaculatory duct obstruction is rare, but is one of the most challenging problems for the urologist[1-3]. The ejaculatory ducts anatomically traverse the posterior aspect of the prostate, entering the prostatic urethra lateral to the verumontanum, just proximal to the external urethral sphincter. These ducts transport the sperm, vasal and seminal vesicle fluid into the posterior urethra during emission.

Obstruction at the distal portion of the ejaculatory duct halting seminal emission may be congenital or acquired. Acquired obstructions are more common, and may be caused by any agent or foreign body which produces severe posterior urethral inflammation[1,2]. Four cases of profound oligozoospermia or azoospermia are presented with diagnostic and management criteria.

METHODS AND RESULTS

Four patients, ages 28, 33, 38 and 40 were evaluated at Duke University Medical Center for profound oligozoospermia or azoospermia from 1974 to 1981, and were found to have sperm counts of less than 5 million on two successive semen analyses over a 2–6 week period. All patients had scant seminal plasma with semen volumes of less than 1.5 ml. Seminal pH averaged 6.8 and seminal fructose was negative in all patients. Diminished semen

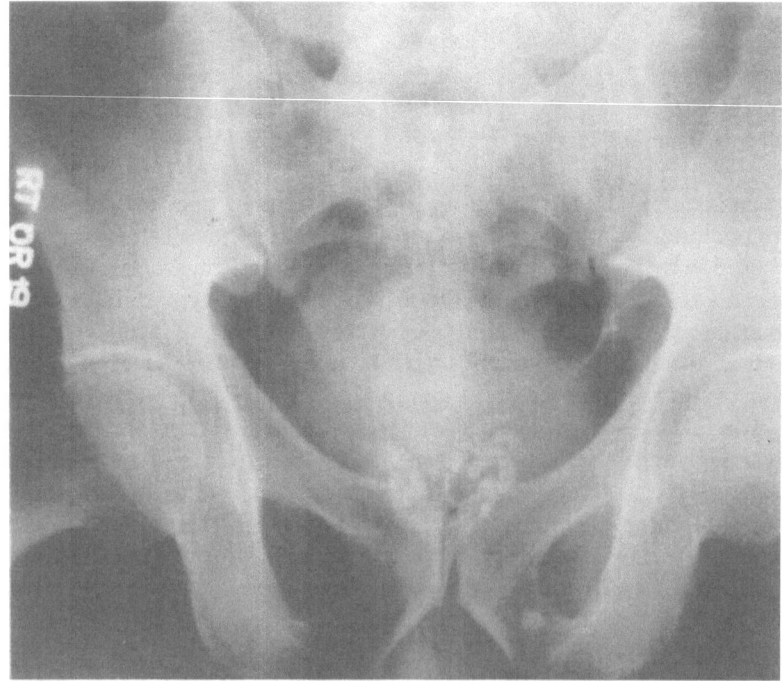

Figure 1   Normal, patent vasogram with efflux of contrast media into the bladder and urethra

Table 1 Results of surgery for ejaculatory duct obstruction

Patient	Age	Diagnosis	Sperm count/Motility ($\times 10^6$)		Semen volume (ml)	
			Pre-Op	Post-Op	Pre-Op	Post-Op
1	28	Indwelling catheter and trauma	Azoospermic	22/55%	0.5	4.5
2	33	Prostatitis/ history of gonorrhoea	Azoospermic	8/25%	0.5	2.5
3	38	Prostatitis/ history of gonorrhoea	2/10%	18/22%	1.0	3.0
4	40	Prostatis	Azoospermic	Azoospermic	1.0	1.5

coagulation was noted in five out of eleven specimens. All patients had normal serum testosterone, LH and FSH levels. Physical examination was unremarkable in two patients, but a boggy, tender prostate was observed in one patient. Past history suggested a longterm indwelling Foley catheter in one patient after severe abdominal trauma following an automobile accident. Two patients had a history of recurrent prostatitis and inflammatory posterior urethritis from gonococcal urethritis prior to the discovery of azoospermia. The remaining patient had only a history of bacterial prostatitis.

Patients were examined in the operating room under general anaesthesia, with subsequent testis biopsy and unilateral vasogram being performed using 5 ml of Renografin 30 mixed 1:1 with sterile saline. Preliminary films revealed prostatic calculi in one patient, but were unremarkable in all others. The criteria for a patent vasal system is visualization of contrast media in the posterior urethra or bladder after injection of 5–10 ml using a 23 gauge scalp vein needle to cannulate the vas deferens (Figure 1)[4]. A distinct obstruction could be seen in all patients, with an end to the column of contrast media at the ejaculatory duct (Figure 2). Repeat films after further injection of contrast

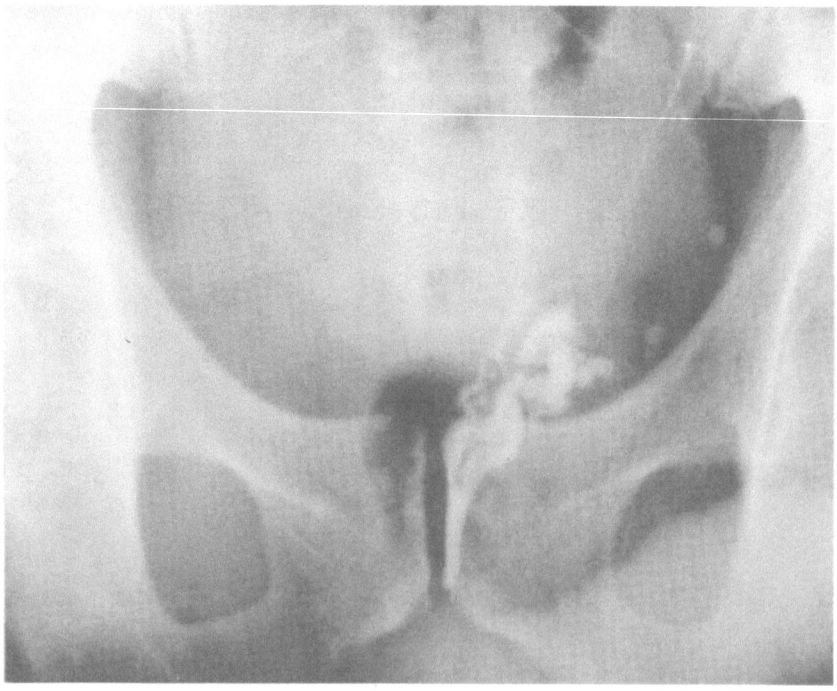

Figure 2 Obstruction of the ejaculatory duct in a patient after urethral trauma from an indwelling catheter and prostatitis

media in all cases confirmed the obstruction of the ejaculatory duct. Testis biopsies revealed normal seminiferous tubules and spermatogenesis in all patients.

Cystoscopic evaluation of the urethra was then carried out, and no fluid was seen effluxing from the ejaculatory ducts in any patients. In the most recent case, 3 ml of indigo carmine diluted 1:4 with saline was injected before cystoscopy, further confirming the complete obstruction visually. Using a standard resectoscope, a small area of the posterior prostate lateral to the verumontanum was resected, taking special care to avoid penetrating the prostatic capsule or injuring the external urethral sphincter. The vesical neck must be carefully preserved to eliminate possible retrograde ejaculation post-operatively. In all cases, contrast medium or indigo carmine could be seen effluxing from the resected ejaculatory ducts. This finding was confirmed radiographically with a repeat vasogram at the time of surgery (Figure 3).

Post-operatively, semen analyses were evaluated monthly for 6–12 months; the longest follow-up was 36 months. Three patients had sperm in their ejaculates initially, with a return of normal ejaculatory volume and fructose

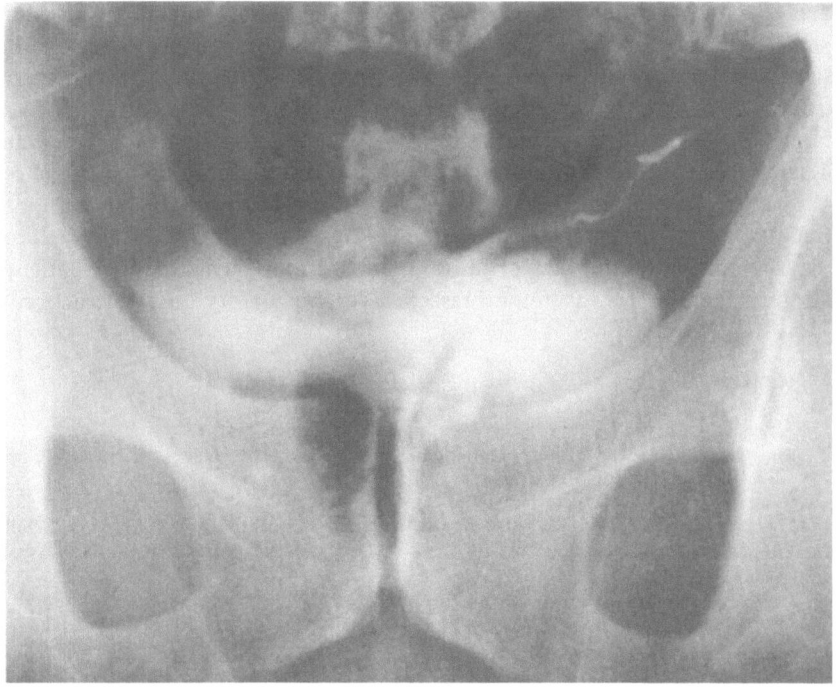

Figure 3 Normal ejaculatory duct patency after transurethral resection

content. One patient remained azoospermic after verumontanum resection despite a patent vasogram. Sperm counts, however, were restored to fertile levels in only one patient with post-Foley catheter obstruction. This patient's counts varied from 15 to 25×10^6/ml, with 55% motility. Two remaining patients had counts varying from $4-18 \times 10^6$ ml with motility varying from 10 to 25%.

DISCUSSION

While infertility and azoospermia caused by bilateral ejaculatory obstruction is extremely rare, vasography performed at the time of testicular biopsy can easily reveal those patients with this intriguing condition. Causes of ejaculatory obstructions include inflammatory conditions such as prostatitis, tuberculosis and gonococcal urethritis. Urethral trauma, longterm indwelling urethral catheters, urethral foreign bodies or transurethral surgery can also produce ejaculatory duct obstruction.

While restoration of fertility after transurethral resection of ejaculatory ducts is unlikely, probably secondary to epididymal blow-outs or re-stenosis, return of even minimal sperm transport may allow future artificial insemination or in vitro fertilization. Surgical resection, however, must be carried out with great care to avoid post-operative complications such as retrograde ejaculation, incontinence or re-stenosis of the ejaculatory ducts. Frequent failures to restore fertile semen specimens in our series and others probably results from stenosis beyond the level of the verumontanum from chronic inflammation[1]. It should be noted that our successfully treated patient had an obstruction related not to chronic inflammation, but probably to the local trauma of a urethral catheter. Despite the low success rate of this procedure, the low morbidity and lack of other treatment modalities for these patients supports the use of transurethral resection for ejaculatory duct obstruction.

References

1. Amelar, R.D. and Dubin, L. (1982). Ejaculatory duct obstruction. In Garcia, C., Mastroianni, L., Amelar, R.D. and Dubin, L. (eds.) Current Therapy of Infertility, pp. 80–2 (Trenton, NJ: B.C. Decker)
2. Pomerol, J.M. (1978). Obstructions of the seminal duct. Int. J. Androl. (Suppl. 1), 50
3. Wagenknecht, L.V. (1982). Obstruction in the male reproductive tract. In Bain, J., Schill, W. and Schwarzstein, L. (eds.) Treatment of Male Infertility, pp. 221–48. (New York: Springer-Verlag)
4. Ford, K., Carson, C.C., Dunnick, N.R., Osborne, D. and Paulson, D.F. (1982). The role of seminal vesiculography in the evaluation of male infertility. Fertil. Steril., 37, 552

38
Results of microsurgical testicular autotransplantation in nine patients with high-lying undescended testes

H. GARIBYAN, F. W. J. HAZEBROEK, J. C. MOLENAAK
and N. F. DABHOIWALA

SUMMARY

Extensive initial laboratory experiments in animals have led us to believe that autotransplantation of the testis in the human, using modern day micro-surgical techniques is feasible. To date nine children with undescended intra-abdominal testes have undergone autotransplantation to bring the testes into the normal scrotal position. Using microsurgical techniques we have anastomosed the testicular vessels to the inferior epigastric vessels, and have been successful in bringing every testis down into the scrotum. Patient age varied from 4–13 years, and no post-operative complications have been noted. Post-operative follow-up varies from 9–18 months, and no atrophy of the testes has been observed in this period. Follow-up Doppler investigations on all the transplanted testes continue to demonstrate a good arterial flow.

INTRODUCTION

Approximately 9% of cryptorchid testes are located intra-abdominally or are high-lying in the inguinal canal[1].

In these cases conventional surgical methods will not always enable the testis to be brought into the scrotum.

Since the turn of the century several operative techniques to try and solve

197

this problem have been reported. Some of the better known are: the two-stage orchidopexy and the division of the spermatic vessels (Fowler–Stephens).

Although in a number of cases good results have definitely been achieved with these techniques, the number of abortive attempts leading to testicular atrophy are considerable. A review of the post-operative results in our hospital following the division of the spermatic vessels produced frightening statistics. Testicular atrophy had resulted in four out of eight patients within 6 months of surgery.

In 1976 Silber and Kelly[2] published an alternative procedure. They described the autotransplantation of an intra-abdominal testis using micro-vascular surgical techniques. Subsequently, other authors have also reported success using this method[3-5]. Interest in organ and tissue transplantation has increased dramatically in the last few years, and microsurgical techniques have advanced so rapidly that it is now possible to anastomose satisfactorily blood vessels with a diameter of 0.5 mm. These developments prompted us in our department to attempt similar vascular anastomoses in laboratory rats. Initially, we experimented by cutting the carotid artery transversely and re-anastomosing it end-to-end.

As our operative skill increased we carried out successful anastomoses of the femoral artery, which in the rat is of a much smaller calibre. The femoral vein was also re-anastomosed in a similar fashion; because, unlike the artery, the vein has extremely thin walls. Having obtained sufficient technical expertise we proceeded to experiment with orchidopexy in dogs using the same micro-vascular techniques[6-8].

MATERIALS AND METHODS

In our clinic, nine patients with unilateral intra-abdominal testes in the age range from 4 to 13 years were operated upon. Depending on the position of the testis, the testis can be approached either intraperitoneally or retro-peritoneally. The testis, epididymis, vas deferens and testicular vessels are first inspected, and the testicular vessels dissected free, proximally to the level of the lower pole of the kidney, from the surrounding structures. The epigastric vessels are isolated next, and the vein and artery are cleanly divided under the operating microscope. Thereafter the testicular vessels are divided as high as possible and ligated proximally. The testicular artery and vein are anastomosed to the respective epigastric vessels under the microscope, without any tension being present on the anastomosis. The diameter of the testicular vein varies from 0.8–1.4 mm, and of the artery from 0.5–0.9 mm.

The anastomosis is carried out using 10-0 atraumatic interrupted monofilament nylon sutures. The arterial anastomosis is completed first in order to limit the warm ischaemia time to a minimum. In order to obtain a

Table 1 Testicular auto-transplantation results

Patient number	Age at operation (years)	Side	Operation time (hours)	Follow-up period (months) and condition of testis	Doppler control of testicular vessels	Remarks
1	$5\frac{2}{12}$	R	4	18 Normal	+ +	Unsuccessful conventional expl. 2 y ago
2	11	R	4	15 Normal	+ +	Long loop vas
3	$12\frac{8}{12}$	R	3.5	14.5 high scrotal Normal	+ +	Unsuccessful conventional expl. 3 y ago
4	$6\frac{7}{12}$	R	4	12.5 Normal	+ +	
5	$11\frac{3}{12}$	R	3	12 indurated sperm cord	+	
6	$9\frac{8}{12}$	L	3	12 Normal	+ +	
7	$9\frac{3}{12}$	L	2.5	11 high scrotal Normal	+ +	
8	$3\frac{5}{12}$	L	3	10.5 Normal	+ +	
9	$10\frac{4}{12}$	R	2.5	3 Normal	+ +	Contra-lateral atrophic testis after earlier orchidopexy with ligation of testicular vessels

proper intrascrotal testis it is sometimes necessary to mobilize the vas deferens together with the surrounding peritoneum up to the posterior aspect of the bladder. The testis is fixed in the usual manner in a subcutaneous pouch. Details of the patients have been summarized in Table 1. In seven out of the nine patients the inguinal canal had already been explored prior to the testis transplantation, and the testis identified as lying proximal to the internal inguinal ring. In two patients laparoscopy was undertaken prior to testis transplantation, and the presence of the testis confirmed. Operative time varied from 2.5–4 hours, and the warm ischaemia time varied from 30–40 minutes in our nine patients.

Patients were immobilized in bed for a day post-operatively, and thereafter they were gradually mobilized. Prophylactic antibiotics were not administered, and no wound infections or other complications encountered. Hospitalization varied from 5–7 days.

RESULTS

Nine intra-abdominal testis units in nine patients were transplanted using microsurgical anastomosis techniques. Testicular vessels were anastomosed to the inferior epigastric vessels. Using these techniques all testes could be brought down into the scrotum. During the follow-up period, lasting from 10–18 months, no atrophy of the testis has been encountered. However, in two patients a high scrotal testis is present as a result of a short vas deferens, and in one patient residual induration of the spermatic cord is present 12 months post-operatively.

The testicular vessels are regularly checked by Doppler flow techniques, and proper pulsations are recorded every time.

CONCLUSION

The aim of surgery on the undescended testis is not only to increase the chances of fertility at a later date, or to diminish the possibility of malignant transformation, but perhaps more importantly in the modern world of today to allow these youngsters to have a normal psycho–sexual development as well.

The procedure of testicular autotransplantation with microvascular anastomosis is feasible, and the immediate results appear to be good but we have to await the longterm results.

Our experience has convinced us that this procedure has a greater potential for success than vascular pedicle division alone or a staged orchidopexy.

Microvascular techniques require considerable training and expertise. Consequently, testicular autotransplantation will probably have to remain the prerogative of specialized surgical centres.

References

1. Scorer, C.G. and Farrington, G.H. (1971). *Congenital deformities of the testis and epididymis.* (London: Butterworths)
2. Silber, S.J. and Kelly, J. (1976). Successful autotransplantation of an intra-abdominal testis to the scrotum by microvascular technique. *J. Urol.*, **115**, 452–4
3. MacMahon, R.A., O'Brien, B. McC., Aberdeen, J., Richardson, W. and Cussen, L.J. (1980). Results of the use of autotransplantation of the intra-abdominal testis using microsurgical vascular anastomosis. *J. Pediatr. Surg.*, **15**, 92
4. Giuliani, L., Carmignani, G., Belgrano, E. and Puppo, P. (1981). Autotransplantation de testicules dans la cryptorchidie. *J. d'Urol.*, **87**, 279–81
5. Upton, J., Schuster, S.R., Colodny, A.H. and Murray, J.E. (1983). Testicular autotransplantation in children. *Am. J. Surg.*, **145**, 514–8
6. Garibyan, H. (1981). Experimental microvascular surgical orchidopexy. *Neth. J. Surg.*, **33**, 119–22
7. Garibyan, H., Baumans, V., Klopper, P.J. and Wensing, C.J.G. (1984). Effect of experimental microvascular orchidopexy on spermatogenic cell differentiation in the testes of the dog. *Urol. Int.*, **39**, 21–4
8. Garibyan, H., De Jong, F.H., Klopper, P.J. and Van Der Molen, H.J. (1983). Effect of experimental microvascular orchidopexy on testosterone secretion in the dog. *Urol. Int.*, **38**, 337–9

Section 6

Artificial Insemination

39
Echosonographic control of follicular growth in heterologous therapeutic insemination (AID)

V. RUÍZ-VELASCO, O. B. DE LA PEÑA, E. D. DOMVILLE
and E. M. ZELAYA

INTRODUCTION

Many studies have shown the usefulness of echosonography (ESG) to evaluate the development of ovarian follicles, as well as their rupture during ovulation. The procedure has been used for this purpose in women with normal cycles, patients receiving clomiphene or human gonadotropins in order to induce ovulation, and especially in studies of *in vitro* fertilization[1-4]. ESG has also been used to control patients subjected to artificial insemination by donor (AID), a method which we call heterologous therapeutic insemination[5] (HTI).

Among other measures aimed at increasing the number of successful treatments in the shortest period[6,7], during the last 2 years we have adopted ESG as a routine method of following follicular development in patients subjected to HTI.

The purpose of this paper is to determine the advantages of ESG on the basis of our experience in the most recent series of women who achieved pregnancy by means of HTI.

MATERIAL AND METHODS

Twenty-five patients who achieved pregnancy by means of HTI form the basis of this report. ESG was performed daily or every other day as soon as cervical mucus became evident, or from the 12th day of the cycle when the quality of mucus was poor. Observations were continued until the follicle disappeared or until the next menstrual period when the follicle persisted throughout the cycle. A MultiScan MS 50 Kontron real time apparatus with 3.5 MHz transductor was used.

According to our working routine, most patients received medication to induce ovulation[6,7]. Clomiphene was given in 15 cases, hMG–hCG in one and bromocriptine in three (Table 1). Fresh semen was used for inseminations following the technique of the cervical cup as modified by our group[6,7].

Table 1 Follicular development in cases of pregnancy achieved by HTI

Case number	Cycle with pregnancy		First cycle		Second cycle		Treatment
	MD	DO	MD	DO	MD	DO	
1	21×18	14×12	26×22	18×16			Clomiphene
2	20×20	17×16	20×20	20×17			Clomiphene
3	22×20	13×12	16×16	12×12			Clomiphene
4	20×20	20×20	14×12	14×12			Clomiphene
5	18×17	12×11					Clomiphene
6	22×18	20×18					Clomiphene
7	16×16	16×16					Clomiphene
8	18× 8	18× 8					No medication
9	18×17	18×16	18×16	18×16			Clomiphene
10	27×22	16×14	16×11	16×11			Clomiphene
11	20×18	20×18					No medication
12	20×18	20×18	20×20	10× 9	14×13	14×13	Clomiphene
13	20×18	20×18					Clomiphene
14	20×19	20×19					Bromocriptine
15	22×20	22×20	20×19	11× 9			Clomiphene
16	25×23	25×23	23×20	21×19			hMG–hCG
17	Negative	Negative					Bromocriptine
18	19×18	19×18					No medication
19	14×13	14×13	20×18	15×15			Bromocriptine
20	20×19	20×19	20×17	20×17	17×17	17×17	Clomiphene
21	20×20	20×20					Clomiphene
22	23×23	23×23	23×22	No break	30×30	No break	Clomiphene
23	18×16	18×16	17×15	17×15			Clomiphene
24	40×36	22×20					Clomiphene
25	17×15	17×15	13×12	13×12	20×20	20×20	No medication

MD Maximum follicular diameters (mm)
DO Follicular diameter at probable ovulation (mm)

In all patients records of basal body temperature and daily cervical mucus score were obtained. In some cases a laparoscopy was performed, and determinations of serum progesterone were done during the second half of the cycle.

RESULTS

Results were analysed considering the maximal development of the follicle during the cycle in which pregnancy was achieved, as well as its size at the time of suspected ovulation. We compared these measurements with non-pregnant cycles from patients who required treatment for more than one cycle to achieve pregnancy.

Eleven patients achieved pregnancy during the first cycle under treatment (44%), ten required treatment for two cycles and four for three cycles.

The maximum average follicular diameter during the cycles in which pregnancy was achieved was 20.75×78 mm and in 85% of the women who became pregnant the follicle was at least 18 mm in diameter. Pregnancy, however, was also achieved in three patients with smaller follicles, and one in whom follicular growth was not detected. The diameter of the follicle on the day when conception probably occurred (estimated according to basal body temperature, cervical mucus score and date of HTI) had an average of 18.41×16.78 mm. In the patients who received no medication to induce ovulation, follicular development was somewhat smaller, and reached a maximum average diameter of 18.5×14.75 mm.

Follicular growth was also smaller during the cycles without pregnancy. The maximum average diameter in these cycles was 18.16×17.77 mm and the diameter at the time of ovulation was 16×15.12 mm.

Only one patient had an abortion which appeared uncorrelated to the degree of follicular development (case 18).

COMMENTS

In order to obtain a greater number of pregnancies in the shortest period of time by means of heterologous inseminations, we have established that, in our centre, all cases for HTI must have an adequate selection of donor with study of spermatic intracervical survival, complete evaluation of the recipient women including laparoscopy in many cases[8], routine induction of ovulation and, lately, evaluation of follicular growth and rupture by means of ESG.

Results presented in this paper are in general agreement with other published data. Thus in 85% of the patients the follicle had a maximum diameter of at least 18 mm during the cycle in which pregnancy was achieved. Other reports indicate that this diameter has been at least 15 mm[1] and at least 18 mm in patients subjected to HTI[5]. On the other hand, we had three patients who achieved pregnancy during cycles when their follicles were smaller, and one in whom pregnancy occurred while the follicle could not be identified.

In our experience ESG is useful for following ovulation in patients subjected to HTI, and increases the number of successful treatments, decreases the time required to achieve pregnancy, avoids unnecessary inseminations when there is no possibility of pregnancy, prognosticate failure when there is lack of follicular rupture, and reduce the cost of treatment.

We conclude that measurement of follicular diameter by means of ESG in women subjected to HTI is a helpful auxiliary method which allows a greater number of therapeutic successes in the shortest possible time. In the current series, pregnancy was achieved following the first attempt in almost half of the cases, thus reducing cost and patient problems.

On the other hand, ESG cannot substitute the use of other clinical parameters which are obligatory in these cases, such as basal body temperature, cervical mucus scores, studies of spermatic survival post-insemination and a complete evaluation of the recipient women.

References

1. Seibel, M. M., McArdle, C. R., Thompson, I. E., Berger, M. J. and Taymor, M. L. (1981). The role of ultrasound in ovulation induction: a critical appraisal. *Fertil. Steril.*, **36**, 573
2. Bryce, R. L., Shuter, B., Sinosich, M. J., Stiel, J. N., Picker, R. H. and Saunders, D. M. (1982). The value of ultrasound gonadotropin and estradiol measurements for precise ovulation prediction. *Fertil. Steril.*, **37**, 42
3. Wetzels, L. C. G. and Hoogland, H. J. (1982). Relation between ultrasonographic evidence of ovulation and hormonal parameters: luteinizing hormone surge and initial progesterone rise. *Fertil. Steril.*, **37**, 336
4. Hoult, I. J., Crespigny, L. C. H., O'Herlihy, C., Spiers, A. L., Lopata, A., Kellow, G., Johnston, I. and Robinson, H. P. (1981). Ultrasound control of clomiphene/human chorionic gonadotropin stimulated cycles for oocyte recovery and *in vitro* fertilization. *Fertil. Steril.*, **36**, 316
5. Marinho, A. O., Sallam, H. H., Goessens, L. K. V., Collins, W. P., Rodeck, C. H. and Campbell, S. (1982). Real time pelvic ultrasonography during periovulatory period of patients attending an artificial insemination clinic. *Fertil. Steril.*, **37**, 633
6. Ruiz-Velasco, V. and Rosas, J. (1976). Nuestra experiencia en la Inseminación en la Pareja Esteril. *Ginec. Obstet. Mex.*, **39**, 363
7. Ruiz-Velasco, V., Domville, E. and Rosas, J. (1978). Inseminación Terapéutica Heterologa con Semen Fresco. *Obst. Ginec. Lat. Am.*, **36**, 361
8. Ruiz-Velasco, V. and Barreda, H. (1982). Role of laparoscopy in heterologous therapeutic insemination (AID). *Int. J. Fertil.*, **27**, 119

40
A comparison of fresh and frozen semen in AID practice

W. H. BLEICHRODT and H. G. MUTKE

Since 1967 artificial insemination by donor has been used in our practice to treat selected patients with infertility due to male sterility. Towards the end of 1982 the 1,000th pregnancy resulting from AID with frozen semen provided a suitable juncture for a comparative study to be undertaken on fresh and frozen semen. During the first 2–3 years of AID practice fresh semen was exclusively employed. Recently treatment tended more and more to the use of cryo-preserved semen for practical and organizational reasons. Fresh semen in-semination poses the difficult problem of trying to prevent the chance meeting of donor and recipient; furthermore the availability of fresh semen could not always be guaranteed and patients coming from far afield were subjected to intolerable stress. Frozen semen has the advantage that the same donor can be used when ovulation is delayed.

The selection of donors in our practice followed the internationally recog-nized principles. When 10 pregnancies have been achieved using the same donor's semen he is not recalled for further donations unless the patient wishes to undergo treatment for a second or third pregnancy. By and large most donors are selected from the medical profession, not only on account of intelligence but also the necessary understanding and responsibility for this method of treatment which such individuals possess.

METHODS

Patients are referred by their local gynaecologist at the optimum time for commencement of treatment. The cycle was monitored by serum FSH, oestradiol and the cervical score. More recently the maturity of the follicle is checked by ultrasound. Ovulation induction with clomiphene citrate, hMG and HCG is only undertaken in exceptional cases. A semen sample is obtained and treated with penicillin to ensure complete eradication of bacteria. For improved motility, experiments with Kallikrein and caffeine have been carried out but these showed no perceptible improvements in conception rates.

Samples of semen for freezing are first examined for morphology and motility, diluted 1:1 with an appropriate cryopreservation media to which penicillin has been added and then subjected to a layering, freezing procedure ensuring optimum crystallization protection. The insemination procedure consisted of placing semen in contact with the cervix by means of a cervical cap. Because of uterine contractions and an increased risk of infection we no longer use the intrauterine or intercervical methods. The latter method is un-physiological; furthermore capacitation of sperm is improved when they remain in contact with cervical mucus. Insemination is commenced 2–3 days before the expected time of ovulation. The comparisons between fresh and frozen semen do not take into account the organic or physiological character-istics of the patients, nor the condition of the uterus and tubes. However treatment may have taken place outside the centre. Psychological factors pertaining to sterility are not examined or included in the statistics. Our investigations merely compare conception rates (birth, miscarriage) in fresh and frozen semen and the number of treatment cycles in relation to the age of the patients. Patients who have discontinued treatment before pregnancy or those still receiving treatment have not been included in the study.

RESULTS

In younger women, up to 25 years of age, there was a higher pregnancy rate with fresh than frozen semen (Figure 1); in cases necessitating a longer duration of treatment the situation was reversed in that frozen semen was more effective when treatment lasted longer than one year.

In the 26–30 year age group similar results were obtained whereby therapy using fresh semen was more successful in the shorter time. The same was true for the 31–35 age group. In older patients (36 years and over) fresh semen was at least 30% more successful than frozen semen. Almost two thirds of preg-nancies were obtained within the first 10 treatment cycles and a third of these in the first three months (Figure 2). Even in the first cycle 11.2% became pregnant from fresh semen and 7.5% from frozen semen. After two treatment cycles there was a pregnancy rate of 23% from fresh semen and 15% from frozen. The average insemination time until the patient became pregnant was 7 months with fresh semen and 9 with frozen. The total birth rate was 46.6% with fresh and 41.5% with frozen. Only one third of patients over 36 years of age became pregnant even when treatment lasted one year. From the age of 40 only 5-6% of women became pregnant.

1,238 children were born including 11 sets of twins; 601 were female and 637 male giving a sex ratio of 49 : 51 (Table 1). The spontaneous abortion rate following insemination with fresh semen was 10.3% and this was significantly below the rate for normally derived conceptions. In all age groups where

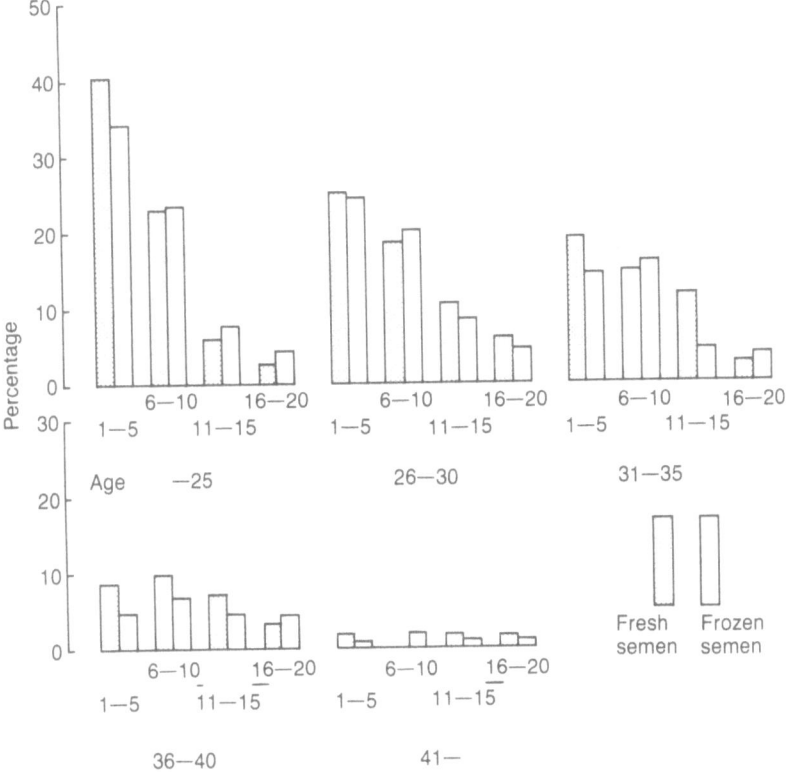

Figure 1 Conception rate in proportion to the age of patients and the number of needed cycles (expressed as a percentage)

frozen semen was used the abortion rate was 2%. This suggests that cryo-preservation results in a favourable selection of sperms. Congenital abnorm-alities in this series were not above normal for the population as a whole; there was a slightly lower rate reported in pregnancies derived from frozen semen but this was not statistically significant.

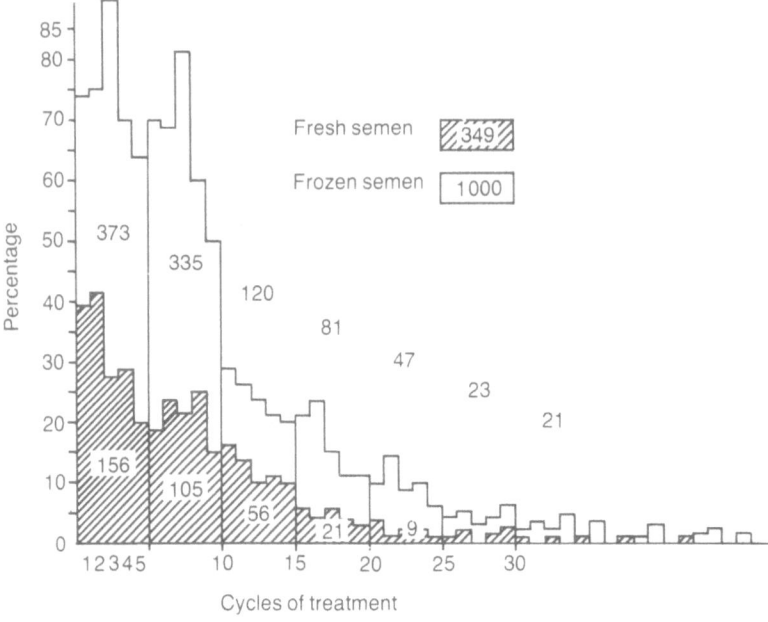

Figure 2 Summary of 1349 conceptions in proportion to the number of needed cycles

SUMMARY

The use of frozen semen for AID is just as effective for achieving pregnancy as fresh semen. It has the added advantage that spontaneous abortion rates in pregnancies from frozen semen are extremely low. It is suggested that freezing of sperm to −190 °C allows only the biologically strongest sperms to survive intact and thereby improves the quality of the semen. Further research is needed to explain why some apparently normal motile spermatozoa cannot be successfully frozen. Even ejaculates from the same donor show inconsistencies in their capacity to withstand freezing.

Bibliography

Barkay, J., Zuckermann, H., Sklan, D. and Gordon, S. (1977). Effect of caffeine on increasing the motility of frozen human sperm. *Fertil. Steril.*, **28**, No. 2, February, 175–77

Beck, W.W. (1976). Modern Trends – A critical look at the legal, ethical and technical aspects of artificial insemination. *Fertil. Steril.*, **27**, No. 1, January, 1–8

Behrmann, S.J. (1979). Artificial insemination and public policy. *N. Engl. J. Med.*, **306**, ??

Belaisch, J., David Georges, Salat-Baroux, J. and Schwartz, D. Spermogramme et Fertilite du couple. *Contracep. Fertil. Sex.*, **6**, No. 11, 767–74

Bergmann, P. and Ullstein, M. (1971). Praxis der heterologen Insemination. *Gynäkologe*, **3**, Heft 4, der Gynäkologe, 159–63

Table 1 AID by a) Fresh semen and b) Frozen semen (summary of 1349 conceptions)

Age		Number of patients	Cycles of treatment	Average	Conceptions n	Conceptions %	Deliveries n	Deliveries %	Abortions n	Abortions %
<25	a	163	646	5.43	119	73.0	109	66.8	10	8.4
	b	306	1546	7.06	219	71.5	204	66.7	15	6.7
26–30	a	176	794	6.97	114	64.7	105	59.6	9	7.7
	b	579	3304	9.03	366	63.2	342	59.1	24	6.5
31–35	a	201	712	7.91	90	44.8	80	39.8	10	11.1
	b	808	3407	10.05	339	41.9	306	37.9	33	9.7
36–40	a	73	227	10.33	22	30.1	16	21.9	6	27.2
	b	280	787	12.29	64	30.7	53	18.9	11	17.6
41–	a	59	57	14.30	4	6.8	3	5.1	1	25.0
	b	226	202	16.80	12	5.5	9	3.9	3	25.0
Total	a	672	2436	6.98	349	51.9	313	46.6	36	10.3
	b	2199	9246	9.25	1000	45.5	914	41.5	86	8.6

from Bleichrodt-Mutke (1983)

Bleichrodt, W. H. and Mutke, H. G. (1981). The present-day position of AID in the Federal Republic of Germany and its practical applications. In *III World Congress of Human Reproduction*, 22–26 March, West Berlin

Bregulla, K. G. (1980). Studies on the storage of human sperm by deep freezing Artificial insemination. *Gynäkol. Praxis*, 4, 243–61

Bromwich, P. et al. (1978). *Br. J. Obstet. Gynecol.*, 85, ??

Campana, A., Gigon, U. et al. (1981). Die Vorbedingungen zur arteficiellen Insemination mit Spendersamen. *Inform. Ärzt*, 3, 26–31

Campana, A., Gürtner, W. et al. (1981). Abortfrequenz und Abortursachen bei Schwangerschaften nach Heterologer Insemination. *Geb. Frauenheilk*, 41, 309–11

Curie-Cohan, M., Luttrell, L. and Shapiro, S. (1979). Current practice of artificial insemination by donor in the USA. *N. Engl. J. Med.*, 300, Nr. 11, 585–90

David, G., Gernigon, C. and Kunstmann, J. M. (1978). Insemination artificielle avec sperme du conjoint. *J. Gynecol. Obstet. Biol. Repr.*, 7, 686–92

Dixon, Richard E. and Buttram Veasy, C. Jr. (1976). Artificial insemination using semen: A review of 171 cases. *Fertil. Steril.*, 27, No. 2, February, 130–34

Friedmann, S. (1977). Artificial donor insemination with frozen human semen. *Fertil. Steril.*, 28, No. 11, November, 1230–33

Gigon, U. (1977). Erfahrungen mit der heterologen Insemination. *Fortschr. Med.*, 95, Jg. Nr. 35, 2124–26

Hellman, R. and Rose, G. (1970). Die heterologe Insemination als therapeutische Maßnahme bei androgen unfruchtbaren Ehen. *Deutsch. Ärtz.*, Heft 13, März, 997–1002

Iizuka, R. (1958). Medical analyses of heterologous artificial inseminations with special reference of frozen storage of human spermatozoa. *Jpn. J. Fertil. Steril.*, 3.1, 359–61

Karow, A. M. College of Georgia School of Medicine anl. der Tagung der American Association for the Advancement of Sciences

Katzorke, T., Propping, D. and Tauber, P. F. (1981). Results of donor artificial insemination (AID) in 415 couples. *Int. J. Fertil.*, 26(4), 260–66

Katzorke, T., Propping, D., Tauber, P. F. (1981). Zyklusstörungen während konsekutiver artificieller Inseminations therapie und ihre Behandlung. *Forts. Med.*, 99, Nr. 13, 471–74

Katzorke, T., Propping, D., Tauber, P. F. and Ludwig, H. (1980). Artifizielle Insemination mit Spendersamen (AID) 140 Schwangerschaften bei 290 Ehepaaren. *Frauenarzt*, 5, 21. Jahrgang, 405–12

Koren, Z. and Liebermann, R. (1975). Fifteen years experience with artificial insemination. *Int. J. Fertil.*, 21, 119–22

Krause, W. (1979). Die heterologe Insemination – Ihre Voraussetzungen und Durchführung. *Inform. Ärzt.*, 5, 92–6

Kupka, H. W. (1981). Die heterologe Insemination in der freien Praxis. *Geburtsh. Frauen.*, 41, 309–11

Lauritzen, Ch. (1981). Die heterologe Insemination. *Deuts. Med. Wochen.*, 106, 195–97

Lübke, F. (1972). Sterilität der Frau – Äthiologie und Diagnostik. *Med. Klin.*, 67, Nr. 25, 867–73

Lübke, F. and Lorenz, E. (1972). Qualtitätskontrolle fertilen und subfertilen Kryosperma unter dem Aspekt therapeutischer Insemination. *Arch. Dermatol. Forsch.*, 244, 447–51

Menkin, M. F., Lusis, P., Zaikis, J. P. Jr. and Rock, J. (1964). Refrigerant preservation of human spermatozoa. *Fertil. Steril.*, 15, No. 5, 511–27

von Milbradt, R. and Jäger-Freitag, S. (1971). Eiweißfreier Blutextrakt (Actihaemyl) als Adjuvans zur Verbesserung der Spermatozoen-Motilität. *Münch. Med. Wochen.*, 4, 142–44

Mochimaru, F. (1979). Artificial insemination with frozen donor semen: its current status and follow-up studies. *Keio J. Med.*, 28, 33–4

Mutke, H. G. (1969). Homologe und heterologe Insemination in der Praxis. *Ärztl. Praxis*, XXI, 5482

Mutke, H. G. (1969). Über Erfahrungen mit der homogenen und heterologen Insemination in der gynäkologischen Praxis. *Presented at the European Congress of Fertility and Sterility*. July. Dubrovnik

Mutke, H. G. (1972). Results in 51 pregnant women following heterologous insemination with semen preserved in nitrogen. *Presented at the European Congress on Sterility.* Month? Athens

Mutke, H. G. (1972). Results in 44 pregnant women following heterologous insemination with semen preserved in nitrogen. *Presented at the VII World Congress on Fertility and Sterility.* Month? Tokyo

Mutke, H. G. (1972). Der heutige Stand der heterologen Insemination. Mitteilungsblatt, Verband der niedergelassenen Dermatologen Deutschlands XX, 56, 17-20

Ockel, G. (1967). Erfahrungen mit der heterologen Insemination. *Deuts. Ärtz.*, Heft 28, 29, 30

Ockel, G. (1967). Zehnjährige praktische Erfahrung mi der therapeutischen heterologen Insemination. *Deuts. Ärzt.*, Heft 28, 29

Ockel, G. (1970). Über zwölfjährige praktische Erfahrung mit therapeutischen heterologen Inseminationen. *Hess. Ärzt.*, Heft 5 Mai

Ockel, G. (1968). Die therapeutische heterologe Insemination - eine dankbare ärztliche Aufgabe. Kleinschriftenverlag G. Ockel Frankfurt

Pedersen, H. and Lebech, P. E. (1971). Ultrastructural changes in the human spermazoon after freezing for artificial insemination. *Fertil. Steril.*, 22, No. 2, February, 125-33

Perloff, W. H., Steinberger, E. and Sherman, J. K. (1964). Conception with human spermazoa frozen by nitrogen vapor technic. *Fertil. Steril.*, 15, No. 5, 501-4

Propping, D., Katzorke, T. and Tauber, P. F. (1981). Further evaluation of the split ejaculate for artificial insemination. *Eur. J. Obstet. Gynecol. Reprod. Biol.*, 11, 385-94

Sato, H., Mochimaru, T. *et al.* (1979). Kallikrein Treatment of Male Infertility. In Editors? *Kinins II: Biochemistry Pathophysiology, (Plenum Publishing Corp.)*, 529-36

Sawada, Y. (1964). The preservation of human semen by deep freezing. *Int. J. Fertil.*, 9, No. 3, July-Sept., 525-32

Sherman, J. K. (1964). Research on frozen human semen - past, present and future. *Fertil. Steril.*, 15, No. 5, 485-99

Sherman, J. K. (1973). Current perspectives - Synopsis of the use of frozen human semen since 1964: State of the art of human semen banking. *Fertil. Steril.*, 24, No. 5, May, 397-412

Smith, K. D. and Steinberger, E. (1973). Survival of spermatozoa in a human sperm bank - Effects of long-term storage in liquid nitrogen. *J. Am. Med. Assoc.*, 223, No. 7, 774-77

Schaad, G. (1970). Heterologe insemination. *Ungeh. Befr. Deuts. Ärzt.*, Heft 10

Schaad, G. (1972). Instrumental heterologous Insemination and its Medical and Psychological Indications. *Physikal. Med. Rehabil.*, 13, Jahrgang, April, Heft 4, 89-95

Schaad, G. (1970). Erfahrungsbericht 1970 über die therapeutische heterologe Insemination in Deutschland - Vortrag auf der XXIII. Tagung der deutschen Gesellschaft für Urologie in Baden-Baden, 27.-31. Okt.

Schaad, G. (1970). Über die therapeutische heterologe Insemination in Deutschland

Schill, W.-B. (1972). Anwendungsmöglichkeiten der humanen Spermakonservierung. *Med. Gegenw.*, 1590-1605

Schill, W.-B. (1972). Humane Spermakonservierung und therapeutische Ausblicke. *Der Hausarzt*, 23, 525-30

Schill, W.-B. (1973). Probleme der homologen und heterologen Insemination aus andrologischer Sicht - Band VII Fortschritte der praktischen Dermatologie und Venerologie 1973 187-95

Schill, W.-B. (1973). Der Einfluß der kryobiologischen Behandlung von Humansperma auf die Aktivität der akrosomalen Protease Akrosin. *Andrologia*, Heft 4, 333-37

Schill, W.-B. (1974). Quantitative Determination of Acrosin Activity in Human Spermatozoa. *Fertil. Steril.*, 25, No. 8, August, 703-12

Steinberger, E. and Smith, K. D. (1973). Artificial Insemination with fresh or frozen Semen. *J. Am. Med. Assoc.*, 223, No, 7, 778-83

Strickler, R. C., Keller, D. W. and Warren, J. (19??). Artificial insemination with fresh donor semen. *N. Engl. J. Med.*, 293, No. 17, 848-52

Tyler, E. (1973). The clinical use of frozen semen banks. *Fertil. Steril.*, 24, No. 5, May, 413-16

Vasterling, H. W. (1971). Die instrumentelle Besamung als Therapie. *Deuts. Hebam. Zeitsch.*, 23, Jahrgang Heft 10, Okt., 12-17

Vasterling, H. W. (1972). Sterilisiert und doch zeugungsfähig. *Deuts. Ärzt.*, Heft 8 vom 24. Februar, 426-7

Weller, J. (1980). Schwangerschafts- und Geburtsverlauf nach 104 erfolgreichen artifiziellen donogenen Inseminationen (AID) mit Nativ- und Kryosperma. *Geburts. Frauen.*, **40**, 269–75

Zimmermann, S. J., Maude, M. B. and Moldawer, M. (1964). Freezing and Storage of Human Semen in 50 Healthy Medical Students. *Fertil. Steril.*, **15**, No. 5, 505–10

41
AID in the problem patient

T. KATZORKE and D. PROPPING

Studies of pregnancy rates achieved by artificial insemination by donor (AID) which are dependent upon reproductive indices in the female may help to determine a reasonable duration of therapy in individual cases. Cervical mucus, ovulatory function, and tubal mechanisms are only a few of the factors crucial to female fertility. The success rate with AID may be elevated by reporting results as the total number of pregnancies in a group, rather than as the total number of women conceiving. A review of recent representative publications in which data could be calculated on the latter basis gives a range of 43% to 63% conception rates[1,2,3]. An US mail-response survey recently reported a mean success rate of 57% (estimated by respondents)[4].

Interpretation of AID data is made difficult because of multiple methods of recording information. Data from patients who drop from therapy after a few cycles should be included in the computation of pregnancy rate/cycle of insemination, but we agree with Dixon and Buttram[5] that 6 months of unsuccessful AID should elapse before an individual is coded as an AID failure. We[6] recorded only 8.5% total pregnancies after the 6th month, compared with the 5% reported by Dixon and Buttram[1] and the 14% noted by Strickler et al.[7].

Another area of confusion revolves around whether success is reported in terms of number of women conceiving or the total number of pregnancies within a group. The former approach gives lower rates but more meaningful information. In this series, 71.5% of the pregnancies occurred by the end of the third cycle. This compares with 63% at 6 months noted by Strickler et al.[2] and 72% in the series of Dixon and Buttram[1]. After the third cycle the slope for occurrence of pregnancy diminishes. This diminution does not take into account, however, the actual rate of pregnancy in each cycle according to the number of inseminations performed, which decreases with each succeeding cycle as a consequence of pregnancy or drop-out. It is apparent that a rate of pregnancy near 10% can be expected between the sixth and tenth cycles of AID. Behrman[8] noted that 94% of all AID pregnancies are achieved by the 12th month. This type of information is helpful in counselling patients. Candidates should be advised that, although pregnancies tend to occur early in the course of treatment, not less than 6 months should be considered time enough for an adequate trial of therapy.

The amount of pre-insemination evaluation necessary with negative female historic and clinical findings presents a dilemma. Where is the balance point between 'wasted' AID and the cost on one hand, and the cost and risk of invasive diagnostic procedures on the other? Our data shows only 46 of 110 laparoscoped patient failures had pelvic findings to explain continued infertility. Our data suggest the prudence of endoscopic evaluation before AID is initiated if a patient presents with a suspect history or if physical examination indicates the possibility of some abnormality. The same procedure is recommended for those clinically normal patients who fail to become pregnant within 3, and certainly within 6 cycles of exposure[6].

Table 1 shows the follow-up of patients who had diagnostic laparoscopy after six cycles.

In the case of normal genital status and tubal patency, in 43% of cases later pregnancy occurred. However, in cases showing pathology after six cycles, only in one third of cases did pregnancy occur after adequate treatment (Figure 1).

Table 1 Laparoscopic diagnosis in 110 patients failing to conceive with six or more AID-cycles

	Number	Pregnant after adequate therapy
Endometriosis	8 (17%)	6 (75%)
Adhesions	14 (30%) ⎫	
Tubal patency decreased	19 (41%) ⎬	(11) (39%)
Tubal occlusion uni- or bilateral	19 (41%) ⎭	
Polycystic ovary syndrome	7 (15%)	(3) (43%)
Leiomyomata uteri	3 (6%)	(3) (43%)

* multiple diagnosis possible
Normal pelvis   64 (58%)
Pathological findings 46 (42%)

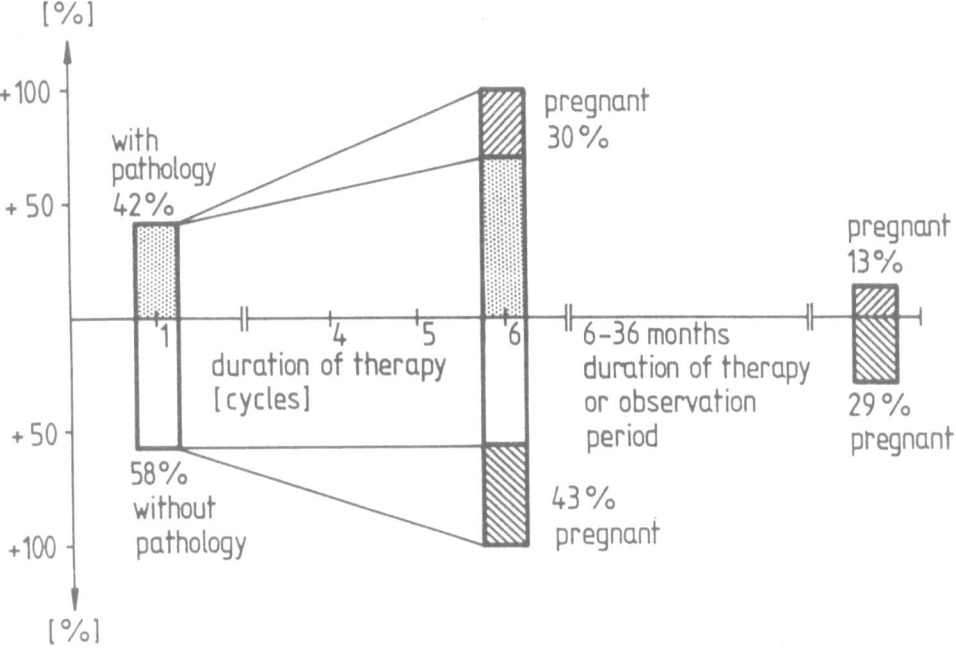

Figure 1

(1) Hysterosalpingography before AID-treatment had only limited value.
(2) Negative laparoscopic findings after six cycles without pregnancy will lead to a pregnancy in nearly 50% of cases.
(3) The incidence of pathologic findings in the pelvis in patients receiving AID is high. In our population it is obvious that abnormalities are found more often as adhesions and occlusions than endometriosis. In the case of pathological findings pregnancy will occur after adequate treatment in about one third of cases.

Our data show a tendency for the number of pregnancies to diminish as age and duration of infertility increase. The variation is slight, however, and we believe that the role played by these factors is minor, although the phenomenon has been documented by others dealing with the general problem of infertility. Schwartz and Mayaux[9] noted an impairment of fertility in the group of patients over 30 years of age, and our findings support this thesis. Furthermore, the abortion rate increases significantly over the age of 35.

Increasing irregularity of the menstrual cycle during AID, especially persistently late ovulation, explains the low pregnancy rate after more than six unsuccessful insemination cycles. Since the pregnancy rate after AID is highest in the first insemination cycle[5,6], it is proposed that ovulation timing, without previous expanded hormone analysis which only delays the treatment, should be started after 2-3 unsuccessful insemination cycles to eliminate possible stress-induced conception failures. After nine unsuccessful insemination cycles one should not hesitate to use hMG/hCG to increase the pregnancy rate.

It must be stressed that the study was retrospective and subject to many of the problems of analysing such data. However, the information gained may aid the clinician in his approach to candidates for AID. The most critical points revealed by the survey are as follows:

(1) Age and length of infertility appear to be of importance in determining the outcome of AID in patients older than 30 years.

(2) Of those patients conceiving, the majority will do so within three cycles of exposure, and 90% will have done so within six cycles of exposure.

(3) An adequate trial of AID therapy should last at least 6 months.

(4) Although the frequently reported conception rate of up to 70% may be expected in patients with correctable ovulation disorders or with normal reproductive organs, a marked diminution in the success rate should be expected in candidates with disorders such as endometriosis, tubal disease, pelvic adhesions and uterine abnormalities.

Although a complete work-up on each patient is not feasible, or even necessary, we believe that the patient should be made aware that predicted rates of success vary greatly, and depend largely upon the degree of selectivity employed in choosing candidates for AID. When given sufficient information, patients with their physicians can plan an approach to AID which may prevent much of the mental, physical, and financial burden of a prolonged (possible futile) regimen of insemination. On the basis of our findings we suggest that the most important factor in success with AID is persistence. Patients should be advised that their chances of conception with AID approaches that of normal fertile couples.

References

1. Bergquist, C. A., Rock, J. A., Miller, J., Guzick, D. S. and Wentz, A. C. (1982). Artificial insemination with fresh donor semen using the cervical cap technique: a review of 278 cases. *Obstet. Gynecol.*, **60**, 195

2. Corson, S. L. (1980). Factors affecting donor artificial insemination success rates. *Fertil. Steril.*, **33**, 415

3. Glezerman, M. (1981). Two hundred and seventy cases of artificial donor insemination: Management and results. *Fertil. Steril.*, **35**, 180

4. Curie-Cohen, M., Luttrell, L. and Shapiro, S. (1979). Current practice of artificial insemination by donor in the United States. *N. Engl. J. Med.*, **300**, 585

5. Dixon, R. E. and Buttram, V. C. (1976). Artificial insemination using donor semen: a review of 171 cases. *Fertil. Steril.*, **27**, 130

6. Katzorke, T.H., Propping, D. and Tauber, P.F. (1981). Results of Donor artificial insemination (AID) in 415 couples. *Int. J. Fertil.*, **26**, 260
7. Strickler, R.C., Keller, D.W. and Warren, J.C. (1975). Artificial insemination with fresh donor semen. *N. Engl. J. Med.*, **293**, 848
8. Behrman, S.J. (1979). Artificial Insemination. *Clin. Obstet. Gynecol.*, **22**, 245
9. Schwarz, D. and Mayaux, B.A. (1982). Female Fecundity as a function of age. *N. Engl. J. Med.*, **306**, 404

42
Repeat pregnancies with AID

B. N. BARWIN

ABSTRACT

The purpose of the study was to evaluate the success rate .of 60 patients requesting a second or subsequent AID. The reasons for failure to conceive a second pregnancy are presented and correlated with the outcome of the initial pregnancy. Second conceptions occurred after a mean 2.8 cycles in 60% of the patients, compared to a mean of 4.5 cycles in the initial pregnancies. The overall pregnancy rate was 42 pregnancies of the 60 patients treated for six cycles of AI. There were three abortions and one ectopic pregnancy in this series. Explanations are offered for the reduced fertility rates.

INTRODUCTION

The acceptability of artificial insemination with donor semen is now more established and accepted, and has led to a demand for second and repeat pregnancies. This study will evaluate the results of the treatment of 60 couples requesting AID and compare this with the outcome of the initial pregnancy.

MATERIALS AND METHODS

Patients

Sixty women were accepted into the AID programme only after irreversible infertility in the male partner due to azoospermia or severe oligozoospermia (Table 1). At the time of the first insemination the average age of the women was 29.2 and 31.2 for the second pregnancy (Table 2).

Table 1 Male factors in repeat AID

	1st	2nd
Azoospermia	45	48
Oligozoospermia	15	12
	60	60

Table 2 Age distribution ($n=60$)

	Distribution	Mean Age
1st pregnancy	25–36	29.2
2nd pregnancy	28–39	31.2

The mean number of years between the initial pregnancy and the second pregnancy was 1.8.

Donors

The semen donors were under 34 years of age, and had been fully screened prior to being accepted for the AI programme. They were carefully interviewed in order to determine the risk of a hereditary disease. Full clinical examination as well as karyotyping, haematological testing for VDRL were also carried out[1]. All semen was collected by masturbation after 3 days of abstinence, and only sperm counts of 50×10^6/ml or higher, with at least 50% motility were used for artificial insemination[2].

Treatment evaluation

Couples requesting AID were required to make a formal application after consultation and counselling. The female partner was placed on a basal body temperature chart and had a hysterosalpingogram and/or laparoscopic hydrotubation[2,3]. The outcome of the initial pregnancy was compared to the present pregnancy (Table 3).

RESULTS

The overall success rate was 72% (42) (Table 3). The spontaneous abortion rate was 10%, with one ectopic pregnancy. There were 36 full term pregnancies and one Caesarian section (Table 3).

The mean rate of cycles for women receiving AID for the first child was 4.8 cycles and 2.8 cycles for a second pregnancy (Table 4).

Table 3 Outcome of pregnancy

	1st	%	2nd	%
Abortions	6	10	4	10
Ectopic	0	0	1	2
Full Term (N)	48	80	36	86
C/Section	6	10	1	1
Total	60	100	42	100

No S/B or NND

Table 4 Repeat pregnancy with AID

Number of patients	60
Pregnancy rate	42
Mean of cycles	2.8

DISCUSSION

The results of previous AID treatment has been shown to affect success, as indicated by the fewer number of AID couples achieving a second pregnancy[2]. It is of interest that the drop-out rate after six cycles was 5%.

In eighteen of the patients who failed to achieve a second pregnancy, one patient had anovulation cycles and failed to respond to clomiphene. Laparoscopy performed and/or hysterosalpingography in 14 of the patients revealed a tubal factor in three cases (5%); endometriosis in two cases (3.3%); while in 12 patients no endocrine or inflammatory or tubal factors could be found (Table 5).

Table 5 Female factors in repeat AID

	Number	%
Anovulation	1	1.7
* Tubal Factor	3	5.0
* Endometriosis	2	3.3
Unknown	12	20.0
Total	18	30.0

* Laparoscopy
  total number = 60

CONCLUSION

Although successful pregnancy may be achieved with AID, full investigation of the female factor must be undertaken, as a successful outcome of an initial pregnancy does not ensure a successful outcome in a second pregnancy.

References

1. Barwin, B. N. and Beck, W. W. (1976). Artificial Insemination and Semen Preservation. In Hafez, E. S. E. (eds.) *Human Semen and Fertility Regulation in Men*, p. 429. (St. Louis: Mosby)
2. Cryglik, D. G., Mayaux, F. and Schwarta, D. (1979). Results of AID for first pregnancy and succeeding pregnancies. In David, G. and Price, W. S. (eds.) *Human Artificial Insemination and Semen Preservation*, p. 211. (New York: Plenum Press)
3. Corson, S. L. (1980). Factors affecting donor insemination rates. *Fertil. Steril.*, **33**, 415

43

The post-insemination test in predicting the outcome of artificial insemination with husband's semen

S. FRIEDMAN

INTRODUCTION

Artificial insemination with the husband's semen (AIH) is frequently performed when there is no apparent cause for infertility other than oligo-asthenospermia or consistently poor PCTs despite normal semen analyses. A test to determine the efficacy of AIH would be helpful to avoid prolonged and possibly futile attempts at conception by this means.

MATERIALS AND METHODS

Sixty three women undergoing AIH for the above indications, had a post-insemination test (PIT) to see if such a test would be of prognostic value. After determining that cervical mucus was adequate, fresh semen obtained from the husband was analysed for concentration and motility. (Morphologic examination was usually done on the first specimen only, obtained at the couple's initial visit, and not at the time of subsequent AI.) A volume of 0.5–1.0 ml was inseminated. A small amount was placed in the cervical canal, some of which invariably spilled back into the vagina, and the remainder in a cap which was then fitted over the cervix. Two to 4 hours later, the cap was removed, cervical mucus was aspirated and examined. This interval was selected based on studies by Tredway et al.[1], who had shown that sperm concentration in the cervical mucus reaches its maximum about 2.5 hours after insemination. Cycles were excluded if the cervical mucus showed a sharp decline in the

227

interval between insemination and PIT. Also, patients were not included in the study if sperm counts were consistently less than 10×10^6/ml, or motility was consistently less than 25%. Preliminary studies had shown that PITs were uniformly very poor or negative in such instances and pregnancies rare by AIH.

RESULTS

The 63 patients were divided into two groups, 13 in Group A who conceived during the study, and 50 in Group B who did not conceive during the study. Table 1 gives the indications for AIH. Oligoasthenospermia was defined as a sperm concentration of less than 40×10^6/ml, or motility less than 50%. What constitutes a poor PCT is controversial. We used less than five motile sperm/high power field (hpf) from 1–12 hours after intercourse as our criterion for a poor PCT. 'Empiric' meant at the patient's request, regardless of the semen analysis or PCT. The incidence of poor semen analyses was the only significant difference between groups. Table 2 compares prior fertility and additional infertility factors, and there were no significant differences here. Endometriosis was treated in all cases, and those with post-operative pelvic adhesions underwent lysis of adhesions. These patients were all laparoscoped sometime before or during the study, except those who conceived during the first 4–6 cycles of AIH, and four patients in Group B. The latter might have had additional factors, but even so, these would not have made a significant difference.

Table 1 Indications for AIH

| | Group | |
	A	B
Oligoasthenospermia	1	14
Poor PCTs	11	33
Empiric	1	3

Table 2 Prior fertility and additional infertility factors

| | Group | |
	A	B
Additional factors:		
endometriosis	2	13
post-op adhesions	2	1
anovulation	1	4

Figures 1 and 2 compare the results of the PITs between the two groups. Figure 1 shows the number of sperm/hpf. The shaded bars represent the group that achieved pregnancy, the clear bars the non-pregnant group. In post-coital testing, there is general agreement that good tests, whether it is the mean of 13 live sperm noted by Moghissi[2] or the 20 or more sperm reported by Jette and Glass[3], are associated with good fertility. Poor PCTs, with less than five sperm, are associated with poor fertility. With post-insemination testing, there was no difference in the distribution of the values between the two groups. Pregnancies occurred despite very poor PITs, and these PITs followed inseminations of semen specimens which were quite representative for these men. They did not follow unusually poor specimens. Figure 2 shows the percentage of motile sperm found on PIT, and again there was no difference in the distribution of the results between groups. Using 50% motility as the dividing line, there was still no significant difference. The number of sperm and the motility usually ran parallel except for two instances in Group B where

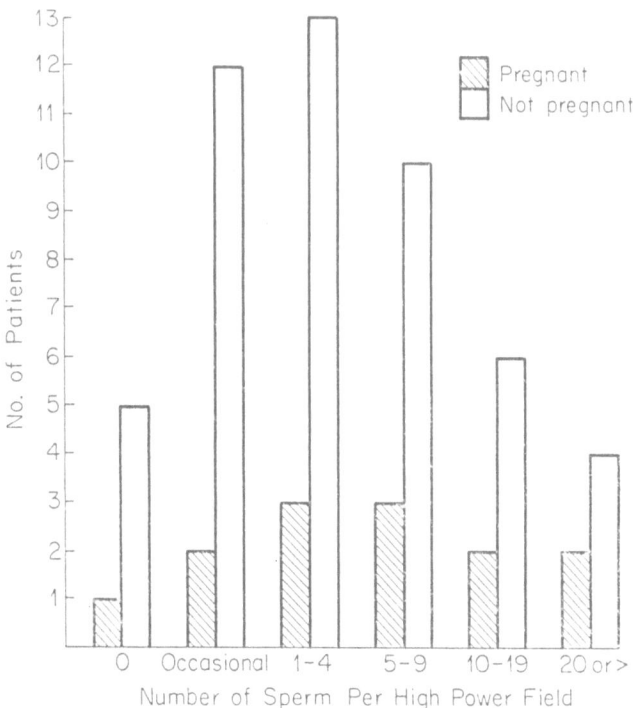

Figure 1 A comparison of number of sperm found on PIT between pregnant and non-pregnant patients

229

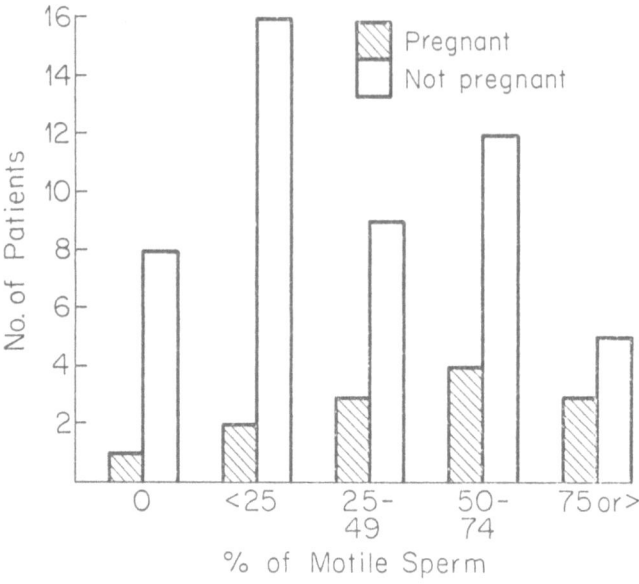

Figure 2 A comparison of the percentage of motile sperm found on PIT between pregnant and non-pregnant patients.

20 or more sperm were found but they were all dead. In these instances, there was probably an immunologic factor in either the cervical mucus or semen.

Six of the 13 conceptions occurred immediately following insemination and PIT, and these cycles were analysed to see if the inseminates or the PITs had any features that would characterize them as likely to be associated with a conception cycle. Table 3 gives the counts and motilities of the inseminates which resulted in pregnancies, and the PITs after these inseminations. There was nothing striking in the semen specimens except that no pregnancy occurred with a poor specimen. As for the PITs, the distribution of the counts

Table 3 PIT in cycle of conception

Semen parameter		PIT parameter	
density (10⁶/ml)	Motility (%)	Sperm/hpf	Motility (%)
100	55	> 20	75
70	40	1–4	50
80	75	5–9	50
70	35	1–4	33
55	75	1–4	25
100	40	5–9	50

and motilities was no different than those just shown on the two bar graphs, except that there were no pregnancies when fewer than 1-4 sperm per high power field were seen, or when motility was less than 25%. However, there were not enough pregnancies to determine if these findings were significant. Three pregnancies occurred after what we would consider a poor PIT, that is, only 1-4 sperm/hpf, two after an equivocal PIT with 5-9 sperm/hpf, and one after a good PIT.

Table 4 compares sperm counts and motilities between groups. All semen specimens were included in the calculations, and since some patients had many more cycles of insemination than others, the results are not equally weighted for each patient. In any case, the mean sperm count was significantly higher in Group A, although motility was not different between groups. Because of the great variation of counts and motilities in the same patient, the ranges were then examined. The figures shown in Table 4 are the range of all the counts of all the patients. The only apparent difference here is the lower range of the counts in the non-pregnant group. As Table 5 reveals, when a determination was made of the number of patients whose lowest counts were under 10 million, it was found that there was a significant difference between groups. Only two of the 13 men whose wives conceived ever had counts this low, whereas 19 in Group B did. Additionally, at the other end of the range, 12 out of 13 men in Group A had counts at one time or another of 80×10^6 or better, whereas only 29 in Group B ever achieved this concentration, and this too was significant.

Table 4 Density and motility of sperm in pregnant and non-pregnant groups

	Group	
Semen parameter	A	B
Mean density (10^6/ml)	70.2	46.9
range	27-128	10-127
Mean motility (%)	54.6	62.5
range	23-75	20-84

Table 5 Highest and lowest sperm concentrations

	Group	
	A (n=13)	B (n=50)
Highest sperm count > 80×10^6/ml	12	29
Lowest sperm count < 10×10^6/ml	2	19

In conclusion, this study indicates that mean sperm counts and the range of counts are of greater value in predicting the outcome of AIH, than is a 2–4 h post-insemination test.

References

1. Tredway, D. P., Settlage, D. S. F., Nakamura, R. M., Motoshima, M., Umezaki, C. V. and Mishell, D. R. (1975). Significance of timing for the postcoital evaluation of cervical mucus. *Am. J. Obstet. Gynecol.*, **121**, 387
2. Moghissi, K. S. (1978). Significance and prognostic value of postcoital test. Presented at the *American Fertility Society Meeting*, March 29–April 1, New Orleans
3. Jette, N. T. and Glass, R. H. (1972). Prognostic value of the postcoital test. *Fertil. Steril.*, **23**, 29

44
The relationship between the survival of human spermatozoa in culture medium and pregnancy rate

H. KEY and S. AVERY

INTRODUCTION

It was decided to determine whether spermatozoal survival in culture medium bore any relationship to the number of pregnancies they obtain. It has been observed[1] that the passage of spermatozoa into columns of diluent having a composition similar to tubal fluid yielded sperm with greatly improved motility and survival rates. The chemical composition of the culture medium is based on the electrolyte composition of human tubal fluid and mammalian oocyte culture medium.

METHOD

Aliquots of donor semen were collected (at least three samples). Using a Makler counting chamber, values for its count, motility and progression were obtained; 0.2 ml portions of seminal fluid were mixed with an equal volume of medium. These samples were left for 24 hours at 20 °C and re-analysed. A recovery rate was then calculated for each specimen. Any pregnancy that was achieved was noted against the relevant specimen.

RESULTS

Average recovery rates for each donor specimen ranged from 26.1% to 96.4%.

Pregnancy rates for each donor specimen ranged from 0% to 21%. Figure 1 shows the relationship between the pregnancy rate and the average recovery rate for each donor. Average recovery rates for donors specimens achieving no pregnancies ranged from 26.1% to 72.5%. No pregnancies were achieved with samples when the average recovery rate was <36%. For a specimen to obtain ≥5% pregnancies its average recovery rate had to be > 46%. 51.7% of donor samples analysed achieved 5% or more pregnancies. Out of 19 single sample pregnancies 79% had an average recovery rate of ≥60%.

Figure 2 attempts to determine whether a relationship exists between the

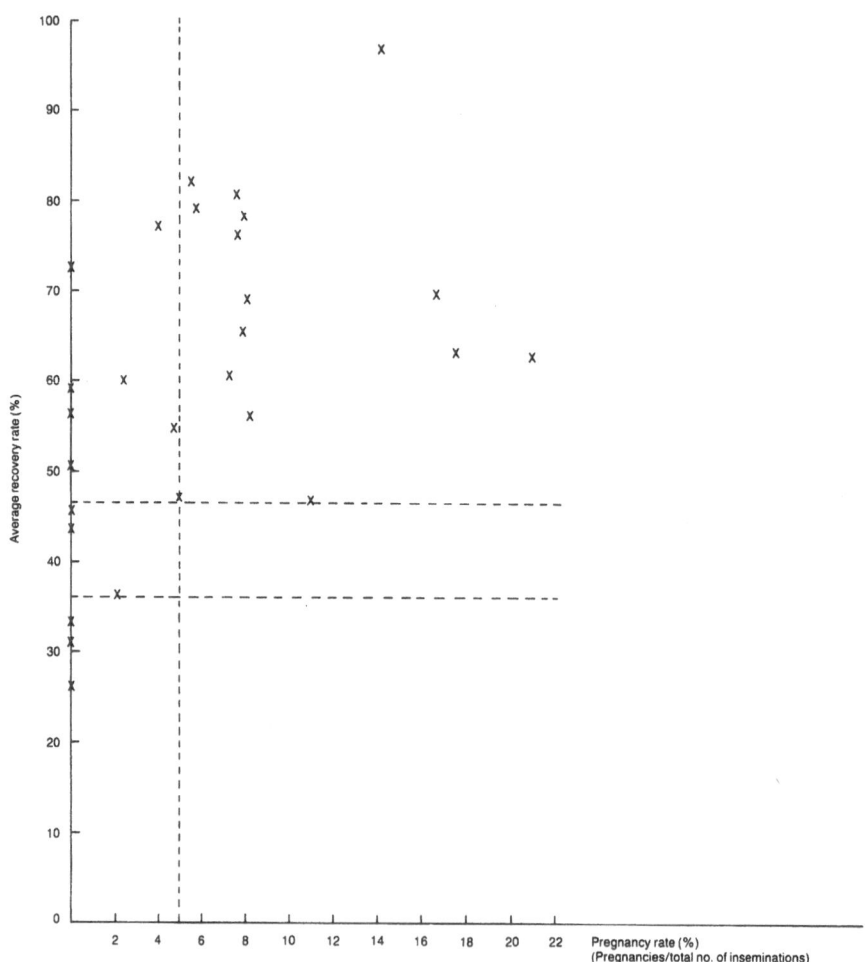

Figure 1   Relationship between pregnancy rate and average % recovery rate of sperm

number of motile sperm in a sample achieving a pregnancy and its recovery rate on that day. No causal relationship was found. However, taking a dividing line at a recovery rate of 45%, 18.75% pregnancies were produced by

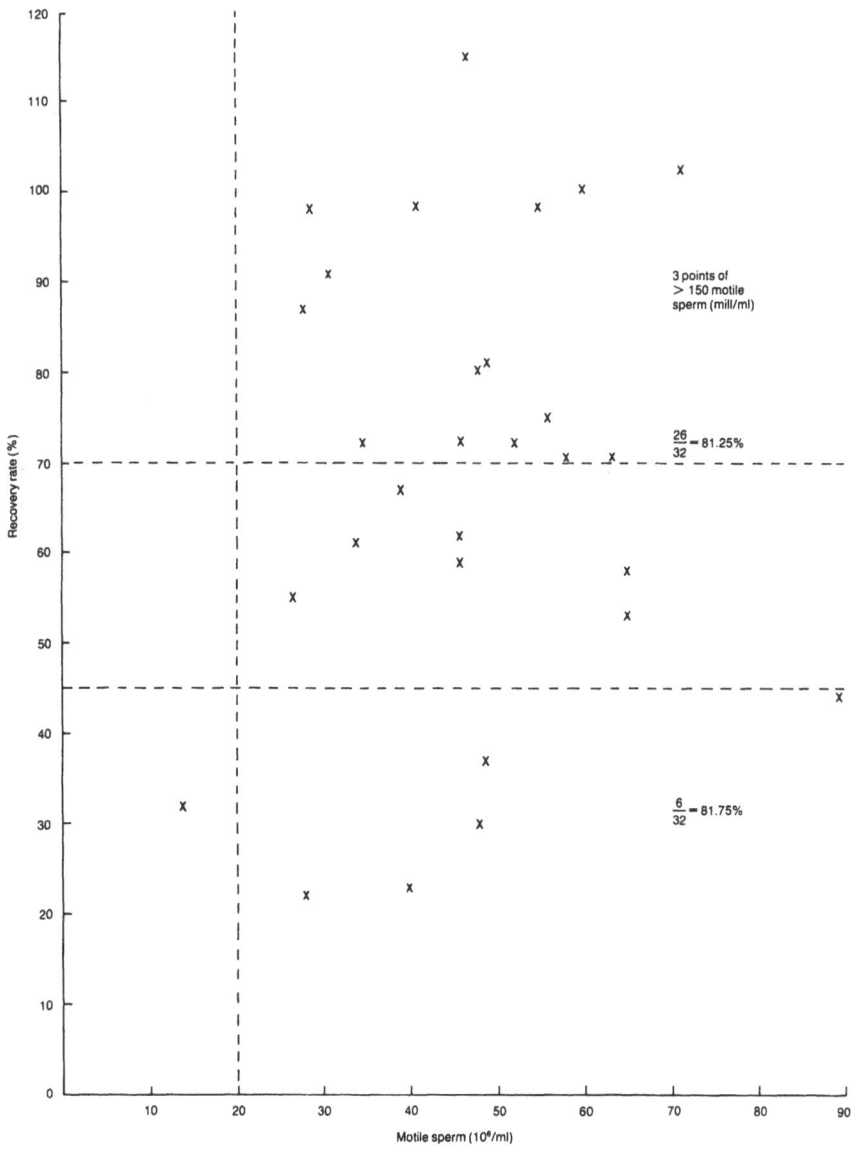

Figure 2 Relationship between motile sperm (10⁶/ml) and % recovery rate

specimens with rates below this, whereas 81.25% occurred with recovery rates greater than this. Seventy-five per cent of pregnancies were produced from spermatozoa achieving a recovery rate of > 70%.

CONCLUSION

Since in this study 79% of pregnancies were achieved with semen with an average recovery rate of ≥60%, it is felt it would be a useful addition to other criteria studied in a seminal analysis.

References

1. Lopata, A. *et al.* (1976). A method for collecting motile spermatozoa from human semen. *Fertil. Steril.*, **27**, 677

45
Duration of vitality and migrating ability of +4 °C cryopreserved human spermatozoa

E. KESSERÜ and C. CARRERE

INTRODUCTION

Preservation of spermatozoa by deep-freezing techniques has been extensively studied[1-3]. In contrast to this, little is known about maintaining sperm by non-freezing cryopreservation, and using the protective properties of the well known egg yolk–glycerol based solutions. This could provide a short term storage method for the improvement of AIH or AID practice, by allowing the repeated use of fractions from the same semen sample, and also a better synchronization of insemination with ovulation. For these purposes it certainly would be a less cumbersome method than deep-freezing. The purpose of the present study was to ascertain how long, under these circumstances, spermatozoa remain unaffected in terms of motility and migrating ability.

MATERIALS AND METHODS

The material consisted of 20 fresh ejaculates from normospermic proven fertile donors. After separating a fresh aliquot (control A), 2 ml of the semen sample was added 1:1 to an egg yolk–glycerol based 'protective' solution[4,5] and centrifuged at 500 r.p.m. for 10 minutes. After removing the supernatant, the sample was fractioned into five test tubes; the first was studied immediately (control B). The remaining four samples were kept in the refrigerator at +4 °C and studied, respectively, after 24, 48, 72 and 96 hours; the samples being pre-warmed to 36 °C.

In each aliquot the following studies were made. *Motility* patterns were quantified in a counting chamber. *Migration* was assessed in capillary tubes containing blood serum. Migration speed (depth) and concentration (density) were quantified at 10, 30 and 120 minutes.

RESULTS

Sperm motility values are shown in Figure 1. There were no differences between controls A and B. At 24 h values already began to decrease without reaching, however, statistical significance. But at 48 h, the diminution of motility was striking, the difference to controls being highly significant. The declination went on through 72 and 96 h. Concerning *in vitro* sperm migration, the results of penetration distances of the sperm into the capillary tube are shown in Figure 2. Here again, controls A and B were identical, and the diminution at 24 h showed no significance (except at 30 minutes). At 48 h,

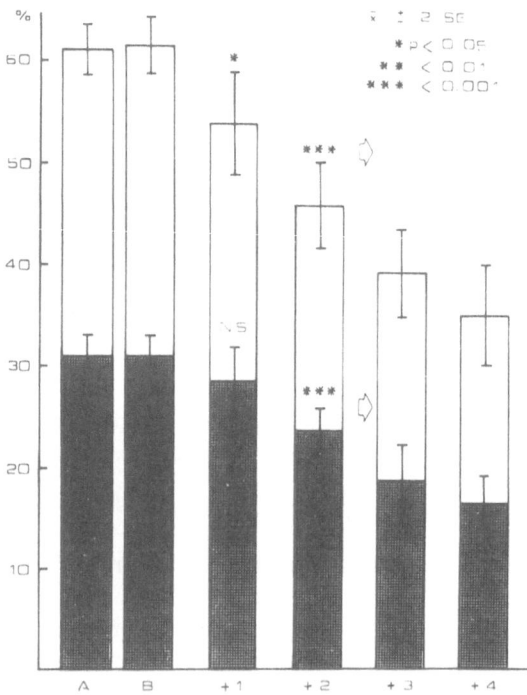

Figure 1 Results of sperm motility light columns present percentages of total motility; dark columns, percentages of sperm with maximal motility.
A = control before resuspending; B = control after resuspending; +1 = after 24 h, +2 = after 48 h, +3 = after 72 h, and +4 = after 96 h of cryopreservation at +4 °C. p values are calculated in comparison to control A ($n = 20$)

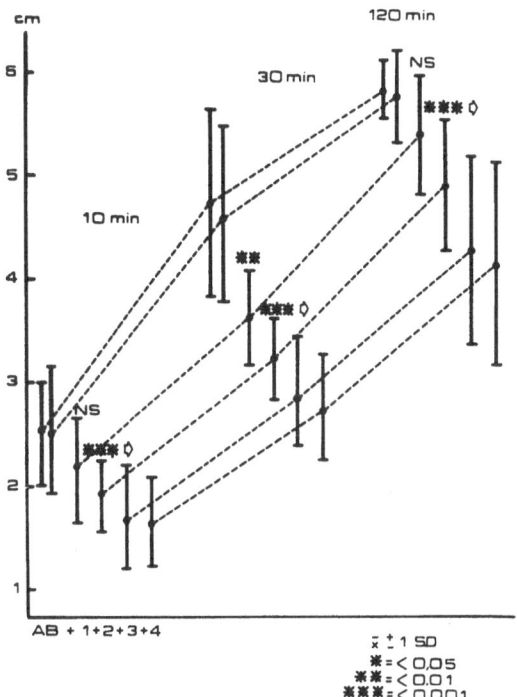

Figure 2 Penetration depth. Figures represent the distances travelled by sperm (±1 SD) into the capillary tubes, after 10, 30 and 120 minutes of initial control. For other details see legends to Figure 1

however, the impairment became very evident, with high significance against controls.

Figure 3 summarizes the results of penetration density. Until 24 h the sperm concentration values remained unchanged. After that time there was a rapid declination, with highly significantly lowered values from 48 h onwards.

DISCUSSION

Only in recent years has there been some evidence that human semen can be stored by a method other than deep-freezing; although, it has been known for 25 years in the case of bull semen[6]. Zavos et al.[7] and Goodpasture et al.[8] demonstrated that motility and acrosin-enzymology of human sperm remains unaffected at $+5\,°C$ until 24 h. Jaskey and Cohen[9] have followed sperm motility patterns up to 96 h, as was done in the present study. We have focussed on both motility and migrating ability in vitro. Human blood-serum was used as the culture medium, in order to keep this variable constant, and because migration patterns are very similar as when using human cervical

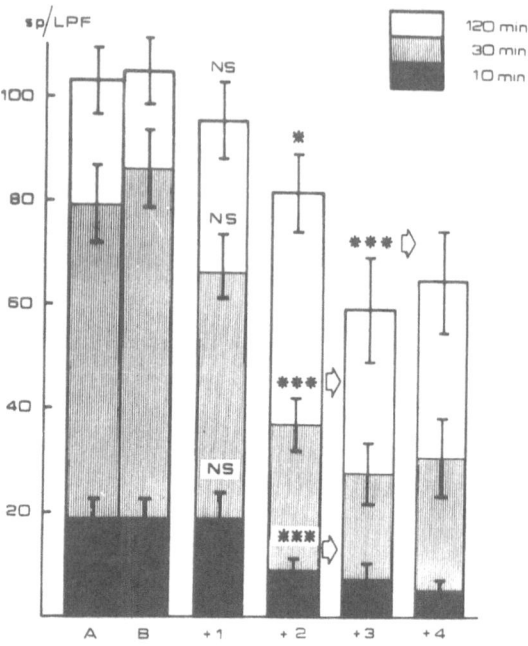

Figure 3 Penetration density. Figures represent the concentrations of sperms per microscopic field (mean ±2 SE) in the capillary tube, at 2 cm distance of the contact point. For other details see legend to Figure 1

mucus[10]. Concerning the results, at first there were no differences whatsoever between fresh and recently resuspended aliquots (controls A and B).

At 24 h preservation some parameters showed a declining tendency: however, without attaining statistical significance. An important finding was that after this time a rapid deterioration began, and at 48 h all parameters were significantly sharply impaired ($p < 0.001$) in comparison to controls. Between 48 and 96 h deterioration went further, though at a slower pace.

The correlation of these laboratory findings with actual fertility still remains to be done. The only conclusion we may draw is that under *in vitro* conditions, the motility and migrating ability of +4 °C cryopreserved human spermatozoa remains intact only up to 24 hours.

References

1. Richardson, D.W., Joyce, D. and Symonds, E.M. (1980). *Frozen Human Semen* (The Hague: Martinus Nijhoff)
2. David, G. and Price, W.S. (1980). *Human Artificial Insemination.* (New York: Plenum Press)

3. Leto, S. and Paulsen, J. D. (1982). Insemination of cryo-preserved semen. In Hafez, E. S. E. and Semm, K. (eds.) *Instrumental Insemination*. pp. 179–87. (The Hague: Martinus Nijhoff)

4. Behrman, S. J. and Ackerman, D. R. (1969). Freeze preservation of human semen. *Am. J. Obstet. Gynecol.*, **103**, 654

5. Nakamura, M. S. and Ramos, R. M. (1975). Frozen human semen – a new technique of conservation. In Campos de Paz, A., Drill, V. A., Hayashi, M. and Schelly, A. N. (eds.) *Recent Advances in Human Reproduction*. pp. 66–69. (Amsterdam: Excerpta Medica)

6. Foote, R. H. and Young, D. C. (1958). Fertility of bull semen stored for one or two days at 5 °C in 20% yolk–citrate–glycine–glucose extenders. *J. Dairy Sci.*, **41**, 732

7. Zavos, P. M., Goodpasture, J. C., Zaneveld, L. D. J. and Cohen, M. R. (1980). Motility and enzymatic profile of human spermatozoa stored for 24 hours at +5 °C and −196 °C. *Fertil. Steril.*, **34**, 607

8. Goodpasture, J. D., Zavos, P. M., Zaneveld, L. D. J. and Cohen, M. R. (1981). Effects of various conditions of semen storage on the acrosin system in human spermatozoa. *J. Reprod. Fertil.*, **63**, 397

9. Jaskey, D. D. and Cohen, M. R. (1981). Twenty-four to ninety-six-hour storage of human spermatozoa in test–yolk–buffer. *Fertil. Steril.*, **35**, 205

10. Kremer, J. (1968). *The in vitro Spermatozoal Penetration Test in Fertility Investigations*. pp. 50–73. (Groningen: Drukkerij van Denderen)

46
Male sterility caused by anejaculation – aetiology, diagnosis and treatment

Z. ZUCKERMAN, Y. TADIR and J. OVADIA

INTRODUCTION

Nonejaculatory intercourse is a complaint encountered in infertility clinics, among childless couples. Masters and Johnson[1] used the term ejaculatory incompetence defined as the inability to ejaculate intravaginally. Retarded ejaculation is a term used by Kaplan[2], for specific inhibition of the ejaculatory reflex. Steeno et al.[3] used anejaculation, to describe the absence of ejaculation, whether by masturbation or during intercourse, although nocturnal emissions do occur. Primary or secondary anejaculation is due to psychological factors that may block or delay orgasm; organic, toxic or mechanical causes are seen to a lesser degree[1-4]. Pelvic operative procedures or spinal cord trauma may damage lumbar sympathetic ganglia and cause anejaculatory orgasm, which must be differentiated from retrograde ejaculation.

MATERIALS AND METHODS

Among couples referred to our infertility clinic during 1981–1982, 12 males desiring to have children presented with symptoms of anejaculation during intercourse.

The mean age was 31 years, with a range of 21 to 40 years. They had been married from 1–15 years (average of 4.75 years). We evaluated the aetiological factors and offered specific individual treatment modalities. Four men presented with combined dysfunction with secondary impotence; four either did not recognize, or denied anejaculatory intercourse. A detailed history of

243

sexual behaviour and basic sex information and education revealed the problem. We performed a comprehensive sexual and genitourinary history, physical examination, hormonal profile including plasma levels of gonado-tropins, testosterone and prolactin. Semen for analysis was obtained by masturbation or collected in a 'Mylex Sheath' at nocturnal emissions.

The differential diagnosis between anejaculatory orgasm and retrograde ejaculation was made by microscopic examination of a post-orgasm centrifuged alkaline urine specimen, for the presence of sperm[4,6].

Treatment included:

(1) Sex therapy[1,2,5] with a multimodal individual treatment approach.

(2) When sex therapy was rejected by the couple or treatment failed, instructions were given for a simple intravaginal artificial insemination using a canula, to be carried out by the couple at home during the ovulatory period. Semen was collected either by masturbation or after nocturnal emissions in the 'Mylex Sheath' special condom[6]. Samples obtained during non-ovulation were deep frozen using liquid nitrogen vapour and glycerol as the cryoprotective agent, then thawed for insemination at the proper time.

(3) Artificial insemination by donor in cases with organic pathology.

RESULTS

In four males the diagnosis was of an organic aetiology for anejaculatory orgasms, with negative findings in urine. One male, aged 23, had undergone left orchiectomy and thoraco-abdominal radical retroperitoneal lymph node dissection for teratocarcinoma of the left testis. Pathology among other patients included congenital megacolon with resection of the sigma loop for bowel obstruction at age 5 years, low back injury at age 12 resulting in fusion of L4–5, spinal fracture with a lesion at L3–4, age 38.

These patients opted for artificial donor insemination, which resulted in three pregnancies.

Deep seated psychogenic factors were revealed in the aetiology of eight patients whose history, physical examination and laboratory tests failed to disclose any organic pathology. Two men presented secondary anejaculation after a specific traumatic event that preceded the acute onset of the dys-function, resulting in fear of coitus and pregnancy, and rejection of spouse. These couples responded to sex therapy and pregnancy ensued shortly thereafter.

Four men were able to ejaculate by masturbation, another four had ejaculation during nocturnal emissions, only. One out of two responded to sex therapy followed by pregnancy. Another two pregnancies were achieved after self-insemination at ovulation with the husband's semen collected by masturbation, and in another case, semen from nocturnal emission was used successfully. Altogether there were six pregnancies in eight cases. There were no positive results with frozen semen obtained by nocturnal emission and inseminated during the ovulatory period.

DISCUSSION

When an organic origin for anejaculation is diagnosed, and post-ejaculatory urine reveals negative findings for sperm, the only treatment available today is AID. Freezing of semen before surgical procedures that may impair ejaculation, should be recommended, but pregnancy cannot be guaranteed.

The most difficult cases for treatment are those who experience only sporadic nocturnal emission[2]. The main contributing factors in the aetiology of primary anejaculatory intercourse in six patients were strict religious orthodoxy with conservative upbringing, three extremely religious men never masturbated. Masturbation is condemned as a grave sin, and is forbidden on the basis of the Talmudic interpretation of biblical verses. An adult male is forbidden to deliberately waste his semen, and deserves the death penalty by strict Orthodox view. Nocturnal emissions that they occasionally experienced caused some men to suffer from guilt feelings and some expressed their wish to control them.

Lack of basic sex education was the cause for anejaculation in five patients. Two patients were surprised to learn that the sexual act means thrusting, while they just used to penetrate and stay still. Suppressed anger and hostility toward a domineering and over controlling spouse, with severe marital conflicts was the source of trouble in three couples. The wives interpreted the husbands inability to ejaculate intravaginally as personal rejection, or felt that they were not sexy enough. Performance anxiety reinforced secondary impotence in three, and hidden homosexuality was disclosed in one patient. Another typical manifestation was long standing erections during sexual activity, up to 30 minutes or more, sometimes until exhaustion, with an insufficient level or almost complete lack of arousal, that never led to ejaculation. Also quite prominent was a lack of pleasure sensations in the penis during intercourse. The ability to attain and sustain an erection in the absence of desire and arousal is a characteristic feature[5].

In sex therapy Masters and Johnson[1] demand strategy with step-by-step assignment of masturbation training: then, the women are trained to stimulate the penis up to ejaculation, with the ultimate goal of intravaginal ejaculation. Since these steps were not acceptable to Orthodox couples, we, therefore, used sex education and information in addition to sensate focus exercises to facilitate self awareness of body sensations. Relaxation training, enhancement of the level of arousal and pleasure sensations, improved communication and exploration of intrapsychic and interpersonal conflicts were recommended therapies.

Most important is the counterbypassing strategy by Apfelbaum[5]. An expressive technique, helps to verbalize worries and sexual feelings, and increases level of arousal. We achieved 75% success rate with sex therapy, a good result compared with other authors[7]. Therapy resulted in three pregnancies shortly after cessation of therapy. If therapy fails, and the only possible way to obtain semen is at nocturnal emission, a 'Mylex Sheath' should be used every night. When nocturnal emission occurs, it can be inseminated. One Orthodox couple succeeded after six repeated trials. Another Orthodox male provided semen sporadically ejaculated at nocturnal emission for freezing, and inseminations at the optimum time, however, as yet there are no results, most probably because of low sperm quality.

Two couples refused to go through intensive sex therapy and asked for artificial insemination. They were under severe pressure exerted by parents, family relatives and peers to conceive as soon as possible. They masturbated, collected the ejaculate and inseminated their wives twice during the ovulatory period in the privacy of their homes. In both cases pregnancy occurred after the first trial. It appears that the longer the dysfunction of anejaculation persists, the less are the chances for successful therapy.

References

1. Masters, W. H. and Johnson, V. E. (1970). *Human Sexual Inadequacy.* pp. 116–36. (Boston: Little and Brown)
2. Kaplan, H. S. (1974). *The New Sex Therapy.* pp. 316–38. (The New York Times Book Co: Brunner Mazel Publication)
3. Steeno, O., Geboes, K. and De Moor, P. (1977). Male impotence: diagnosis and therapy. In Hafez, E. S. E. (ed.) *Human Reproductive Medicine,* 1. *Techniques of Human Andrology.,* pp. 432–3. (Amsterdam: Elsevier – North Holland Biomedical Press)
4. Reckler, J. M. (1983). The Urologic Evaluation of Ejaculatory Disorders. (Male orgasm disorders, RE and PE.) In Kaplan, H. S. (ed.) *The Evaluation of Sexual Disorders: Psychological and Medical Aspects.* pp. 139–149. (New York: Brunner Mazel)
5. Apfelbaum, B. (1980). The Diagnosis and Treatment of Retarded Ejaculation. In Leiblum, S. R. and Persin, L. A. (eds.) *Principles and Practice of Sex Therapy.* pp. 263–96. (New York: The Guilford Press)
6. Smith, K. D. (1978). Achieving pregnancy for men unable to ejaculate. *Med. Asp. Hum. Sexual.,* 5, 84
7. Kolodny, R. C., Masters, W. H. and Johnson, V. E. (1979). *Textbook of Sexual Medicine.* p. 530. (Boston: Little, Brown and Company)

47
Psychological patterns of AID-demanding marital couples

O. TODARELLO, F. M. BOSCIA, G. A. PATELLA, M. W. LA PESA,
F. MATARRESE, L. NATILLA and A. TARANTO

INTRODUCTION

Several authors point out how frequent and dangerous the emotional complications are that sometimes come across in the plain psychiatric pathology of artificial insemination by donors (AID)[1-12]. This risk can be easily understood if one considers the deep emotional and psychological roots that the act of procreating has for women as well as for men. Procreating through the semen of a third person, the donor, can have deep emotional consequences, which not all subjects are able to evaluate, and above all after AID they are not able to accept and integrate the emotional consequences in their emotional life as individuals and as couples.

In order to prevent possible damage to the psychic balance of not only the couple but also the unborn child, several authors agree that it is necessary to precede the AID with an accurate psychological assessment. Some individuals even consider it necessary that such an evaluation should precede the clinical and instrumental investigation, since an eventual contradiction could emerge from the psychodiagnostic study which could make investigations useless[1-4, 6,7,10,12-14].

To obtain a psychological assessment of couples asking for AID different authors have employed various tests and methods; such as M.M.P.I., Rorschach, different rating scales to determinate neurotic and psychotic states, standardized psychiatric conversation, semi-standardized and free conversation. In our experience it has been noticed that the combined use of the normal psychiatric interview, of the Rorschach's test and of the Bellak's test on the ego functions have been found to be useful.

The data from these three different methods are based mainly on different methodological presuppositions but with a common psychoanalytic approach, sensibly reduces the possibility of an incorrect evaluation. The aim of this present communication is to illustrate the data we have obtained with such tests on 20 couples asking for AID.

MATERIALS AND METHODS

Our sample consists of 20 couples who in 1982 asked to be subjected to AID. The women have a mean age of 34.3 years (22–41); the men have a mean age of 33.4 years (26–45). The education level of the women is, 23.8% university graduates, 11% upper school, 17.8% lower school and 47% junior school; for the men the education level is, 17.8% university graduates, 11% upper school, 47% lower school, 23.8% junior school. The couples on the whole have been married for a mean of 6.6 years (1–16).

Each person has been subjected to a series of examinations, gynaecological and andrological which have shown different pathological conditions causing male sterility. Each person was subjected to a psychiatric examination to exclude any possibility of psychiatric disease. Subsequently the patients were given the Rorschach's test and the Bellak's test. The Rorschach psychodiagnostic test was administered by a psychologist as a general projective instrument in his original analytic formulation[15,16].

The Bellak's test, administered by a psychiatrist is based on subjecting the individual to a questionnaire consisting of over 100 questions, divided into 12 groups. Each group of questions concerns a single function. Twelve functions are examined[17]: (1) Reality test, (2) Judgment, (3) Sense of reality, (4) Regulation and control of drive, affect and impulse, (5) Object relations, (6) Thought processes, (7) Adaptation regression in the service of the ego, (8) Defencive functioning, (9) Stimulus barrier, (10) Autonomous functioning, (11) Synthetic-integrative functioning, and (12) Mastery and competence.

The interview is conducted by only one interviewer who records the entire proceeding. Two psychiatrists independently evaluate the results, that is, the allotment of points for every function, from which the mean score is assigned by the two evaluators on a scale of 1–13. For 1–6 points (with a mean of 3) gives the psychotic area, from 4 points to 8 points (with a mean of 6.5) is the borderline area, from 6 to 10 points (with a mean of 8) is the neurotic area and finally from 8 to 13 points (with a mean of 11) is the normal area.

Out of the 20 couples three haven't completed the above-mentioned preparatory programme for AID. For this reason they have been excluded. Therefore, our data refers to the 17 remaining couples.

248

RESULTS

The analysis of the data of the Bellak's test

The information taken from the Bellak's test of the individuals of the 17 couples has allowed us to draw up a graph for each subject interviewed. We then drew up a single graph of the mean numerical values of each single function of the male sample and then, separately, the female sample[17] (Figure 1).

(1) *Reality test*. The two samples show an effective distinction and perception of the internal and external events. The two corresponding sets of numerical data vouch for a medium value within the normal range.

(2) *Judgement*. Occasional errors of judgment are noticed in the male sample showing numerical values within the medium – low limit of the normal range. Whereas the data which refers to the female sample is situated within the medium value of the normal range.

(3) *Sense of reality*. The depersonalization and derealization phenomenon of the two samples is not noticed; the limits of ego are well demarcated with a well constructed sense of self. The numerical data is situated around the medium values of the normal range.

(4) *Regulation and control of drive, affect, and impulse*. There is evidence of the tendency of a little automatic control in conflicting situations and environmental stress. In fact the score gives a medium–low value within the normal range.

(5) *Object relations*. Both of the groups are only sporadically disturbed. The others are perceived as separate individuals and well differentiated from themselves except in stressful situations; sometimes the absence of an emotionally important person is not tolerated. The score is situated in the low area of the normal range.

(6) *Thought processes*. The examined subjects show a certain difficulty in conceptualism and lack of imagination when dealing with objective facts. Such a deficiency is noticed in a more marked way in the male sex. In fact for the men the numerical value is found in the low area of the normal range, while the women obtained medium–low values.

(7) *ARISE*. There is evidence in both groups of the subjects lack of capacity to regress in the service of the ego, from which a scarce adaptive capacity is derived. In fact the obtained score is placed in the low area of the normal range.

(8) *Defencive functioning.* The data from both groups is situated in the medium–low level of the normal range. In fact in the majority of subjects there emerges a note of anxiety and disphoria, in spite of the use of defences mostly in the service of adaptation.

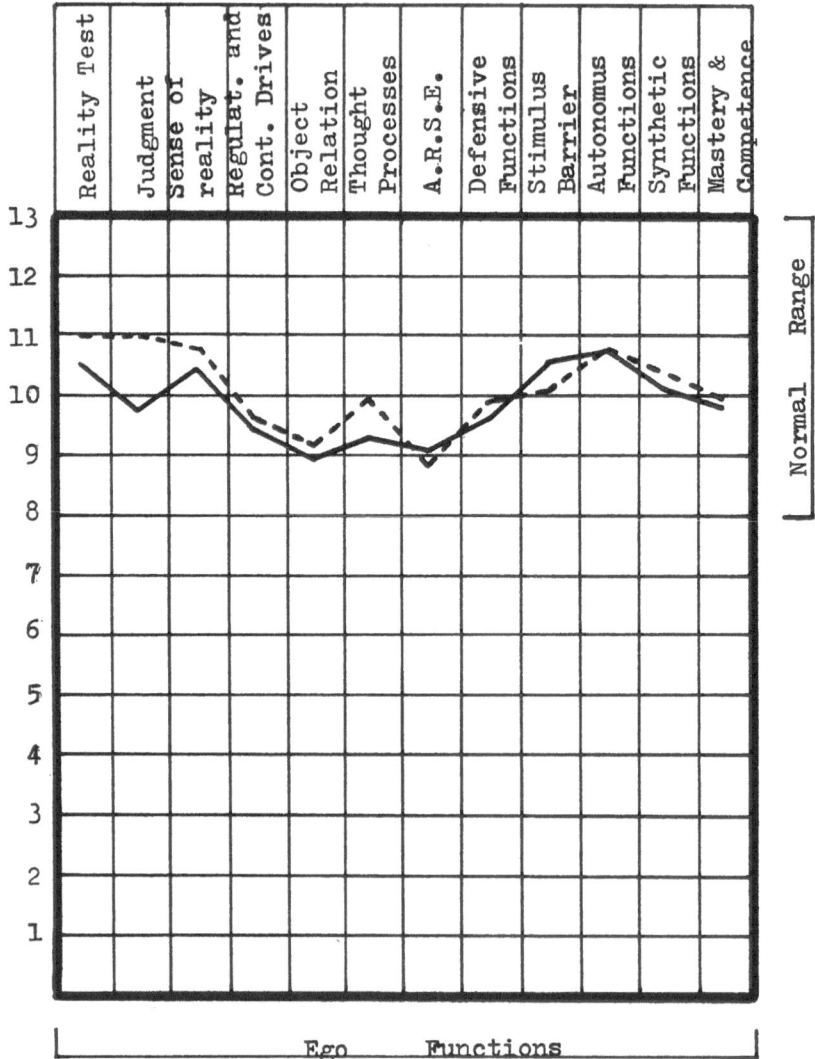

Figure 1 Bellak's test. —=mean values of the male sample; ---=mean values of the female sample

(9) *Stimulus barrier*. The threshold of sensorial stimulation is relatively high; though in the group of female subjects it could be that the focal stimulation disturbs them. The obtained data is around the medium values for the male sample, and around the medium–low values for the female sample, as always within the normal range.

(10) *Autonomous functioning*. The data from the two samples gives medium values within the normal range; the subjects experience a small and sporadic pressure in primary and secondary autonomy.

(11) *Synthetic-integrative functioning*. In both samples a discrete level of integration and coherence is noted in the psychic and behaviour events. This data falls within the medium values of the normal range.

(12) *Mastery and competence*. The data from the two groups is situated in the medium–low values within the normal range. There does not seem to be a considerable discrepancy between the actual competence and the sense of competence.

In examining the above-mentioned graph a notable superimposition is evident in the two curves, which completely falls within the normal range. One can only note small differences between the two samples in the 'Judgment', 'Thought processes' and 'Stimulus barrier' functions.

Analysis of the Rorschach data

The data attained from the Rorschach test show a basic agreement between the male and female samples. Therefore, for the 12 Rorschach functions we have considered in this study we will discuss the male and female together (Figure 2).

(1) *Function G* (The function shows the global perception of the cognitive performance of the subject: this function is connected with function M concerning the strength of ego). It is evident from the data in our possession that the two samples display superior values over the normal range. Pressing conflicts exist, which accelerate this performance.

(2) *Function F* (The function shows the tendency to transform experiences into formally descriptive cognitive elements). The data from the two samples show inferior values to that of the normal range. The subjects find difficulty in expressing their experiences in a descriptive and analogical language.

(3) *Function F+* (The function describes a tendency to give a linguistic

251

denomination to the cognitive aspects of experience, which is socially accepted as significant). The data from the two samples vouch for a value inferior to that of the normal range. The tendency to respond symbolically to the conflicting necessity of the subject rather than the conventional social values.

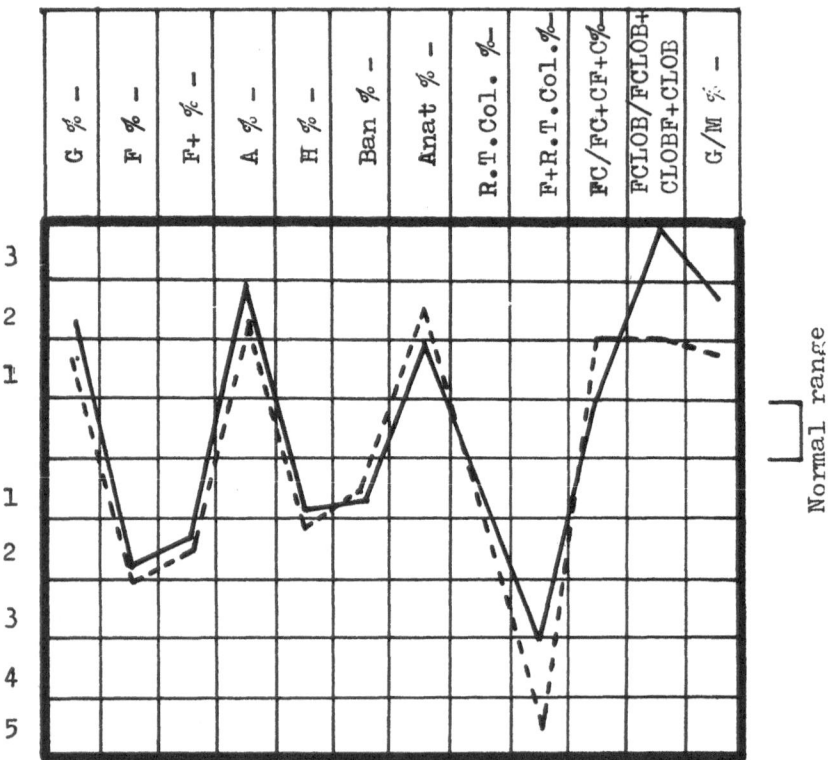

Table 2 Rorschach's test. —=mean values of the male sample; ----=Mean values of the female sample

(4) *Function A* (The function describes the tendency to give 'animal' content to the perception). The data being of equal relevance in both samples, indicates a stereotype superior to that of the normal. The perceptive stereotype seems to be a signal of a marked psychic reality resulting from deep conflicts.

(5) *Function H* (The function describes the tendency to give 'Human'

content to the perception). The data being of equal relevance in both samples, indicates a tendency to remove the interpersonal relationship. This data is found in both of the samples being considered.

(6) *Function Ban* (The function describes the tendency to perceive reality according to a common social standard, in short it emphasizes 'the contact with reality'). In both of the samples this function presents inferior values to that of the normal.

(7) *Function Anat* (The function describes the tendency to give 'anatomical' contents to the perceptions). The values of both of the samples are superior to that of the normal. So there exists a tendency to put into play, in the conflictual reality, the body as an origin of worry. The attention to sexual functions are noted through the body's organs.

(8) *Function R. T. Col.* (The function describes the organic tendency of affective intentionality; where this is minimized one could speak of a tendency towards depression). The data of both samples indicates that a modest inclination exists towards a depressive perception when percepting reality.

(9) *Function F+ R. T. Col.* (The function describes a tendency, with symbolic language, to realize in behaviour, affective intentionality). The data from both samples is lower than that of the normal range. The negativism of affect seems to be a characteristic common to the subjects in our research.

(10) *Function FC/FC+ CF+ C* (The function shows the rigid form or the tendency towards somatization). The relative data of the male sample are within the superior limits of the normal; those relative to the female sample are superior to that of the normal.

(11) *Function FCLOB/FCLOB+ CLOBF+ CLOB* (The function shows the rigid form between the ways of disphoric manifestation). The data of both of the samples are superior to that of the normal. In correlation with 'function 10' in the male subjects this data shows a disturbance even more profound than the need to somatize.

(12) *Function G/M* (The function shows the adequacy characteristic of the ego strength, its capacity to accomplish). The data from both of the samples are superior to that of the normal, the capacity to accomplish the ego is fanciful and without an aim. It is hypertrophic only when confronted with the conflictual immature aspects of ones own experiences.

CONCLUSIONS

Two considerations emerge from the examination of the data:

(1) The examined values of the single functions, in both of the tests, give notably coinciding profiles for both the men and the women (Tables 1 and 2).
(2) The two tests agree significantly when outlining the psychological characteristics of the sample.

In particular the Bellak's test shows a fall in value of the two functions (ARISE and Object Relations) with respect to the others. On the contrary, the values of another three functions (Reality testing, Sense of reality and Autonomic functions) are found in the highest values with respect to those of the other functions.

The Rorschach's test shows an oscillation with respect to the normal range for the G%, A%, Ban, F+R.T. Col., FCLOB functions.

The two tests both point out the fact that the examined subjects have a certain difficulty in adapting to new situations. They are not able to harmonically integrate their own experiences. This is demonstrated in the fall in the value of ARISE in the Bellak's test and also of F+R.T. Col. in the Rorschach's test. In fact the subjects have difficulty in stabilizing a relationship with the outside world, of a formal kind, stereotype, with a scarce affective participation as shown by the elevated values of the functions 'Reality Test' and 'Sense of Reality' in the Bellak's test, and also the A and G functions in the Rorschach's test.

Other confirmations at this time, come from the difficulty these people have in stabilizing really valid relationships with others on an affective level, this is indicated from the oscillation in respect to the normal range of R.T. Col. and G/M functions in the Rorschach's test, and the fall in value of the Object Relations in the Bellak's test.

It is quite uncommon that 34 subjects of both sexes, with different education cultures, present the same homogeneity in psychological characteristics. In this regard, one can formulate two hypotheses:

(1) That the emotions provoked by the sterility problem and by the secrecy that surrounds it induces the ego of these subjects to activate defensive manoeuvres that outline the above-mentioned profile;
(2) That the choice of AID to resolve the sterility problem, in respect to other alternatives such as adoption, is taken mostly by people who have peculiar psychological characteristics.

These are only working hypotheses for further study. The formal adherence to the outside world, and the difficulty in relating to it at a deeper level, the rigidity of the ego of these subjects that renders them almost incapable of creatively confronting new situations, reveals, in our opinion, a weak capacity to evaluate and confront, realistically, AID.

On a practical level, our data induces us to advise preparatory psycho-therapy for AID subjects. The aim of this intervention is to acquire a good relationship with reality, and, therefore, the possibility of clearly dis-tinguishing reality from expectations and fears.

References

1. Aboulkhair, N., Bartoleschi, A. and Boscia, F. M. (1980). Indagini preliminari da eseguire sulla coppia che richiede un I.A.E. In "Inseminazione artificiale umana – Atti del primo seminario internazionale" Bari, 1980
2. Berger, D. M. (1980). Couples' reaction to male infertility and donor insemination. Am. J. Psychiatry, 137, 1047
3. Berger, D. M. (1982). Psychological aspects of donor insemination. Int. J. Psychiatry Med., 12, 49–57
4. Bianchini, A. M., Garofalo, D., Calizolari, E. and Alei, G. (1980). Analisi psicologica della coppia richiedente l'I.A.E. "Inseminazione artificiale umana – Atti del primo seminario internazionale" Bari 1980
5. Cohen, J. (1981). Aspetti psicologici e iatrogeni dell'infertilità. Sessuologia, 5, 385–8
6. D'Elicio, G., Campana, A. and Rech, C. (1980). Consultazione psicologica con le coppie candidate all'I.A.D. "Inseminazione artificale umana – Atti del primo seminario inter-nazionale" Bari 1980
7. Graf, U. and Glander, H. J. (1980). Psychological aspects relating to artificial donogenic insemination (A.I.D.). Zentralbl. Gynakol., 102, 774–8
8. Oliviero, F. A. and Guerrieri, D. (1981). Aspetti psicologici dell'inseminazione artificiale eterologa. Sessuologia, 5, 365–70
9. Pasini, W. (1978). Valutazione critica degli aspetti psicologici dell'inseminazione artificiale eterologa. Sessuologia, 2, 39–42
10. Rosenfeld, D. L. and Mitchell, E. (1979). Treating the emotional aspects of infertility: counseling services in an infertility clinic. Am. J. Obstet. Gynecol., 135, 177–80
11. Schjsman, R., Bettocchi, S. and Boscia, F. M. (1980). Inseminazione artificiale umana. "Atti del primo seminario internazionale" Bari 1980
12. Watters, W. W. and Sousa-Poza, J. (1966). Psychiatric aspects of artificial insemination (donor). Can. Med. Assoc. J., 95, 106–13
13. Curie-Cohen, M., Luttrel, L. and Shapiro, S. (1979). Current practice of artificial insemination by donor in the United States. N. Engl. J. Med., 300, 585–90
14. Rutledge, A. L. (1979). Psychomarital evaluation and treatment of the infertile couple. Clin. Obstet. Gynecol., 22, 255–60
15. Exner, J. E. (1969). The Rorschach system. (New York: Grune and Stratton)
16. Rorschach, H. (1947). Psychodiagnostik. (Berne: Verlag Hans Huber)
17. Bellak, L., Hurvich, M., Gediman, H. K. (1973). Ego functions in schizophrenics, neurotics and normal: a systematic study of conceptual, diagnostic and therapeutic aspects. (New York: Wiley and Sons)

48
The complexity of psychological issues involved in artificial insemination by donor

R. ROWLAND

This paper will present an overview of current issues, focusing on the experiences of potential AID parents. Interviews and questionnaire work with over 50 couples at the Melbourne Family Medical Centre in Australia forms the basis for the discussion. In our pro-natalist society, pressure to have children is strong. All people assume they are fertile, and hence it is a shock if one is told that this assumption is false. There is a kind of superstitious belief that infertility is 'somehow meant to be', which can lead an infertile couple to feel they are being punished. Society has taught people that to parent is good, and is a measure of maturity and adulthood[1]. Couples may feel that their pass into adulthood has been denied.

The process of discovering infertility involves unpleasant tests to the point at which the individual feels physically invaded[2]. Women are usually tested first as if it is assumed the infertility is her 'fault'. This leads to resentment when the husband is found to be infertile, and a sense of guilt in both partners. The male feels that it is unusual that he is infertile, and that he is the only man to ever have experienced it.

The process of testing can last from 12 months to 7 years in some cases, involving a continuous cycle of frustration, despair, raised hopes and depression. There is also seemingly endless waiting. These apply stress to the marriage[3]. The initial reaction of the couple to the news of infertility is shock. It has been likened to grief, in that it involves anger, disbelief, frustration and guilt. The loss is that of the kind of biological family now unattainable, and for the sense of the self as a procreative being. The generativity which makes people want to create something or someone to live after them, is usually satisfied through childbearing and rearing, and this initially seems blocked. The self-image is battered and couples experience a loss of personal control in their lives.

Loneliness is a dominant experience at this time. Men are socialized not to express their emotions, particularly those involving vulnerability. This, coupled with their guilt, makes it impossible for many men to discuss the issue on any but a superficial level. The wife is also isolated. She is involved in the mechanistic side of AID, controlled by blood tests, temperature charts and insemination appointments. Her continual travelling, the difficulty of getting time off work, and the unpleasantness of the testing process itself, cannot be discussed easily with her partner. She feels unable to complain about a process which is both desired and disliked. Couples thus often find it difficult to openly discuss the real issues involved, and to make a clear and informed decision about using AID.

A number of guidelines emerge here which are useful in discussion with couples. The man should accept his infertility and develop a self-image not based on procreation through biological parenting. There will always be periods of regret and reassessment as this is a process, not a final static state of mind. Similar processes occur for parents and childfree people: trigger events motivate thoughts of the 'path not taken'[4].

A new definition of sexuality is needed, not based on the biblical concept of sex for procreation alone. In some instances, the couple's love-making fades or ceases altogether because they see no purpose in it. This can lead to a lack of self-esteem, a feeling of being estranged and unloved.

A new understanding of parenting is also needed. A 'baby' tends to become the major aim, and couples should consider a broader definition of child-rearing. A concept of a 'parent' as being one who cares for and rears a child should replace the idea of father and mother equalling biological parents. This involves a move away from the concept of 'ownership' of children.

A great deal of secrecy surrounds AID and this may create a number of problems. Secrecy is usually intended to protect either the AID father or the child. But unless a more positive discussion of AID and its advantages and dis-advantages takes place, attitudes will continue to be negative. It is the infertile man who should be educating the community.

The child's supposed reaction should he/she discover his/her origin encourages parents to deceive the child and hide this information. The assumption is that if they do not tell the child, he/she will not find out. How-ever, most of the couples tell someone, whether it be sister, brother or mother. The possibility is, therefore, always present that under stress one partner or the confidant might break the secrecy. This would be most likely to happen during stressful life-periods, e.g. adolescence or the death of a spouse. Deception of the child will increase stress on the couple and could affect the marriage. This is apart from the issue of the right of the child or any adult to know of their origins, neglect of which can lead to genealogical bewilderment[5]. Furthermore, it intrudes on the rights of *all* children and thus adults, because all children from now on will doubt their parentage. No parent will be able to prove parentage to their child via birth certificates, as these are fraudulent in the cases of donor sperm and donor ova. Distrust will be built into the relationship between all parents and all children unless the legal situation with respect to birth certificates is corrected.

But whether parents intend to tell the child or not (about 50% each way in this study to date), a major problem exists. There are no scripts for explaining the situation. Most people find it difficult to discuss sexuality with their children, and this is one step removed. Even if they do tell of the origin of birth, because of the secrecy surrounding donors they cannot give the child any useful non-identifying information. It is also very difficult for many couples to acknowledge the donor as a man, preferring to see the insemination itself as a medical solution, like a 'penicillin jab'. This fantasy of a non-person solution is designed to protect husband and wife psychologically from the intrusion of a shadowy third person, but may create difficulties when the child is told or finds out the truth.

The AID offspring are currently discussed in relation to the adoption model, where recent changes and increased understanding have led to adopting parents being told to tell the child, while young, of their origins. They are provided with information on the birth parents. Unfortunately, the AID child is always discussed as a 'child' by parents and professionals, which has led to an infantalization of offspring. It enables people to discuss their 'rights' from the superior viewpoint of an adult, and to decide 'what is best' for the child. We should not neglect the fact that AID children become adults with all the complexity of social and psychological experiences that this entails. They may in fact have similar experiences to those adoptees who seek their hidden parents, and research indicates that in one study 60% of donors would be happy to meet with their offspring to discuss family background as long as no legal claims were made on them[6].

From this discussion it is clear that counselling services should be offered to couples from the period involving infertility testing. But there are other instances when it is also needed. If a woman miscarries or if she does not become pregnant, she will feel she has 'failed' in the last chance she had. Her failure will be the worse for having assumed her fertility after her husband's inability. To have completed the whole process and still be childless is a devastating blow to the couple. But currently, these people are left to return to the population and to their lives with no attention or counselling. We have no information on how they cope[7].

Few follow-ups have been conducted on the state of marital happiness after the birth and growth of the AID offspring. A return rate for a second or third child does *not* indicate that the issues discussed here have been resolved. In one follow-up of 50 couples, 'no major obstetric, paediatric or emotional problems were apparent' to the researchers. However, in the same paper they commented that '*all* wives were anxious about their husband's reaction to the child' and 'some problems with interpersonal relationships in the family unit have been encountered'[8].

The medical profession should not be expected, or indeed have expectations itself, which place upon it the burden of dealing with these issues, as well as with the physical aspect of treatment. For self-protection they either assume an air of 'coldness' or become personally stressed at the distress of couples. Regular 'coldness' or become personally stressed at the distress of couples. Regular counselling, which involves some amount of time and experience, should be offered to couples and donors in AID programmes by medical social workers or psychologists, so that doctors are relieved of stress, and couples have all their needs adequately catered for. The result will be a sense of security with respect to the wellbeing of both couples and AID offspring, ensuring the continuation of programmes in a psychologically healthy environment.

References

1. Nijs, P. and Rouffa, L. (1975). AID couples: psychological and psychopathological evaluation. *Andrologia*, 7, 187–94
2. Mazor, M. (1979). Barren couples. *Psychol. Today*, 12, 101–12
3. Bonython, A. (1977). Facing decisions in an artificial insemination by donor programme. *Aust. Child Fam. Welfare*, 2, 47–51
4. Rowland, R. (1983). Childfree and parenting experiences. (In preparation)
5. Sants, H. J. (1964). Genealogical bewilderment in children with substitute parents. *Br. J. Med. Psychol.*, 37, 133–41
6. Rowland, R. (1983). Attitudes and opinions of donors on an AID programme. *Clin. Reproduct. Fertil.*, 2, 13–23
7. Channel 7 (1983). We do know of a suicide of one 'failed' IVF parent in Melbourne: *Last Chance*, 5th June, Melbourne
8. Clayton, C. and Kovacs, G. (1982). AID offspring. Initial follow-up study of 50 couples. *Med. J. of Aust.*, 1, 338–9

49
Secrecy in the provision of artificial insemination by donor (AID)

R. SNOWDEN

Since the first recorded case of AID the practice has grown steadily. The technological aspects of AID have been researched and progress made – for example, in the successful freezing and storing of semen, and in methods of identifying the time of ovulation. Administrative procedures regulating the storage and classification of semen have also been improved. But very little is known of the longterm social and psychological ramifications of this technically simple procedure, and in 1983 we still remain largely unaware of the ways in which AID affects the complex network of family relationships.

SOCIAL ROLES AND AID

The family is the basic unit of social organization in all cultures, and is, therefore, of great importance. The web of family relationships is far more complex than is often supposed, and the implications of these relationships are far reaching. Relatives believe they have ties with each other from which arise rights, duties and obligations; these are grounded in the often unspoken expectations we each hold about the behaviour of other family members. It is not just how an uncle or a father sees his role as uncle or father, but also what others expect of him in that role. These expectations are based on an understanding of the part each of us plays within the family, and are closely related to behavioural predictability. One firm expectation within marriage is that each partner is expected to have a sexual relationship with their spouse and with their spouse only. Of course this expectation is not always met, but it nevertheless persists. It is upon this expectation of exclusive sexual relationships within marriage that the whole rationale of AID is based. AID is not a medical treatment; it does nothing whatsoever to cure a man's infertility – it 'treats' his fit, fertile wife instead. AID does not meet a medical need (that of curing infertility) but a social need of curing childlessness. It does this by introducing fertile semen without a personal, physical relationship, thereby maintaining the social expectation that sexual relationships within marriage should be exclusive. A strictly medical justification for a doctor's involvement in AID provision is difficult to identify. The insemination technique is simple, and women have been known to perform it successfully on a do-it-yourself basis. The main reason for a doctor's involvement appears to be that the doctor acts as an 'honest broker' mediating between the couple and a suitable donor, and also legitimizes a controversial procedure.

SECRECY AND AID

Throughout its development the provision of AID has traditionally been surrounded by secrecy. This secrecy has at least three components relating to:

(1) The confidentiality of the consultation between the doctor and the infertile couple;
(2) The anonymity of the donor; and
(3) The pretence by the couple that the AID child is the result of a natural conception.

The confidentiality of the medical consultation is essential, and there would seem to be good reason for maintaining the anonymity of the donor; conflicting emotional ties between the family of the recipient and the family of the donor would be undesirable. It is the third component of secrecy – the purposeful misleading of close family members, and indeed the child itself – which gives rise to social concern. If family relationships are to function well, mutual trust is an essential ingredient, and this implies an assumption of honesty and truthfulness. Where AID is undertaken secretly and deliberately hidden from some family members, the basis of that trust on which family relationships are essentially built is being undermined.

The assumption of most AID practitioners that secrecy is preferable and beneficial has generally been accepted without question from the earliest days of AID provision, but the reasoning which lies behind this attitude has never been made explicit. The uncertainty of the legal position in most countries has undoubtedly contributed to this perceived need for secrecy, but despite the lack of clear legal support practitioners have exhibited greater confidence in providing an AID service as the procedure has become more widespread, and has taken on a semblance of medical respectability. Secrecy is sometimes justified as being necessary in order to protect the child. Perhaps most often secrecy is justified simply because it is possible, and it allows the couple to appear 'normal'. But this stance of secrecy also has disadvantages; it restricts the availability of information to couples who could themselves benefit from AID if only they knew enough about it. Secrecy means that pressure is not put upon the legal system to institute the necessary legal changes, nor is pressure put upon health service policy-makers to provide adequate finance for clinics. Secrecy implies there may be something shameful about AID, something which cannot be talked about and should be hidden for fear of arousing disapproval. But most importantly secrecy serves to deceive the child about its own identity and genetic history, and undermines the basis of trust on which all family relationships are founded.

To most men knowledge of their infertility comes as a profound shock. Because men hide their infertility each man affected feels that he is the only one so afflicted. Male infertility is often mistakenly confused with impotency and lack of virility, and there is a poor understanding of the meaning of male infertility. Following discussions with approximately 70 couples who are parents of AID children, it emerged that the main reason underlying secrecy is the fear of both the husband and wife that the infertile husband will be stigmatized, that his standing in the eyes of other people will be reduced because of his infertility. In the present climate of general public misunderstanding about male infertility, the secrecy that surrounds AID and the desire of the couple to hide their infertility is understandable, but it is counterproductive. To deal with a problem by denying that it exists rarely produces a satisfactory resolution of the problem. The psychological costs of maintaining a life-long secret are high. Rather than encouraging the denial of the husband's infertility by assuring the couple that 'no-one need ever know', energies should be directed towards establishing an enlightened understanding of the concept of male infertility through education and counselling. The stresses which infertile couples have to face should not be aggravated by a perceived need to hide their misfortune.

Not all couples keep AID secret, and the couples interviewed in a recent study who had decided to tell friends or relatives were glad that they had done so, and had found it helpful. Their confidantes had all been understanding about the situation and had offered wholehearted support and encouragement. Families had all accepted their grandchildren, or nieces or nephews, without reservation and 'thoroughly spoiled' them. The number of AID children who are aware of their different conception is small. The reactions of seven young adults who had been told that they were conceived by AID, and reported in a recent study, suggests that not only is it possible to tell an older AID child of his or her origins, but that is is possible to do so without unduly upsetting either the child or family relationships. These young adults had accepted their AID status equably – even proudly – and the family relationships had generally been enhanced. A clear pattern also emerged that the minimal knowledge of the characteristics of the anonymous donor available to these young people had proved helpful. Whilst it would seem necessary to maintain the anonymity of the donor, nevertheless it is suggested that certain information about the donor could be shared with the recipient family which need involve no breach of anonymity; for example, a description of his interests, aptitudes, work, appearance and temperament. This is the type of factual information that many adopted children seek. It is also suggested that a register of donors should be kept so that non-identifying information relating to the donor's medical or family history could be divulged to the recipient family in case of need.

Bibliography

Snowden, R. and Mitchell, G. D. (1983). *The Artificial Family*. (London: Allen & Unwin Counterpoint PBK)

A fuller account of the research project referred to in the above paper is contained in Snowden, R., Mitchell, G. D. and Snowden, E. M. (1983). *Artificial Reproduction: A Social Investigation*. (London: Allen and Unwin)

Addendum to Section 1: Evaluation of the Spermatozoa

50
Relationships between results of post-coital test and parameters of semen analysis

G. B. LA SALA, L. DESSANTI, A. M. S. FOSCOLU,
G. GHIRARDINI and F. VALLI

INTRODUCTION

The post-coital test (PCT) has been a subject of controversy since it was first advocated by Sims in 1866. Opinions on the value of the test in infertility investigations are still divided. Protagonists find the post-coital test a useful monitor of sexual function, an indicator of sperm action, a barometer of periovular hormonal[1] status and a basic screen for the detection of the cervical factor[2].

Antagonists feel its prognostic significance to be almost valueless and little correlation with fertility has been noted[3]. Indeed, in a previous study, a large percentage of infertile patients became pregnant despite persistently poor post-coital test results[4].

MATERIALS AND METHODS

This study compared 100 PCT results with the semen analysis. The case material for our study consisted of 100 couples who consulted us between January and December, 1982 with sterility for more than 1 year.

These couples were subjected to post-coital tests, while the male partner had a semen analysis. We compared the results of the semen analysis with those of the post-coital test. We effected a cervical score by following Moghissi's criterion[5], and the PCT was performed when the mucus score was between 10 and 15.

Table 1 Results of 100 semen analysis

Sperm density (10⁶/ml)		Sperm with motility 3–4 in the 1st hour (10⁶/ml)		Sperm morphology abnormal configuration	
> 20	79	> 20	45	<60%	68
<20	21	> 10 <20	25	> 60%	32
		<10	30		

The sperm analysis was carried out according to Eliasson's criterion[6], while the post-coital test was evaluated according to WHO values[7].

RESULTS

Table 1 shows the results of the 100 spermograms we studied.

In 79 spermograms, the number of spermatozoa exceeded 20×10^6/ml, while in 21 spermograms, it was lower than 20×10^6/ml. We also considered those spermatozoa with 3–4 motility present in the first hour: this value exceeded 20×10^6/ml in 45 cases, was between 20–10×10^6/ml in 25 cases, and was lower than 10×10^6/ml in the remaining 30 cases.

Regarding the morphology of the spermatozoa in our 100 cases, we observed a percentage of anomalous forms of less than 60% in 68 cases, while this number was higher than 60% in 32 cases.

Table 2 shows the results of the 100 PCT tests. These results were good in 57 cases, insufficient in 30 and negative in 13 cases.

If the PCT was negative or insufficient on the first examination, we always repeated the test to confirm this datum, thus excluding the possibility of research errors. From an initial 20 negative PCTs, we were thus able to drop to 13 negative cases while from an initial 46 insufficient PCTs we dropped to 30.

Our research was conducted in order to study the results of PCT as regards sperm quality. We, therefore, tried to eliminate the causes which, at a cervical mucus level, could alter the results of the PCT. Thus we considered the PCT we were able to effect with an ideal cervical mucus value. We compared the results of the 100 PCTs with the number of spermatozoa present/ml (Table 3).

When the number of spermatozoa was higher than 20×10^6/ml, PCT was considered good in 57 cases, insufficient in 18 cases and negative in four cases. Regarding the statistical evaluation of the indicated data, it is important to

Table 2 Results of 100 PCT

Good	57
Insufficient	30
Negative	13

Table 3   Comparison between sperm-density and PCT results

PCT	Spermatozoa (10^6/ml)		Total
	> 20	< 20	
Good	57	0	57
Insufficient	18	12	30
Negative	4	9	13
	$p < 0.0005$	$\chi^2 = 39.6$	

Table 4   Comparison between PCT results and number of spermatozoas/ml with motility 3-4 in the first hour

PCT	Spermatozoa (10^6/ml) with motility 3-4 in the 1st hour			Total
	> 20	$> 10 < 20$	< 10	
Good	41	16	0	57
Insufficient	0	8	22	30
Negative	4	1	8	13
	$p < 0.0005$	$\chi^2 = 62$		

note a statistically significant dependence between the PCT results and the number of spermatozoa/ml.

Table 4 indicates the comparison between the PCT results and the number of spermatozoa/ml, 3-4 motility present during the first hour. When the number of spermatozoa/ml was higher than 20×10^6/ml, the PCT was considered good in 41 cases, insufficient in none of the cases and negative in four cases.

When the number was between $10-20 \times 10^6$/ml inclusive, the PCT was good in 16 cases, insufficient in eight cases and negative in one case. When the number of spermatozoa was lower than 10×10^6/ml, the PCT was considered good in no case, was insufficient in 22 cases and negative in eight cases. There was a statistically significant dependence between the PCT and the number of spermatozoa with 3-4 motility present during the first hour.

Table 5   Comparison between PCT results and spermatozoa morphology

PCT	Spermatozoa with abnormal configuration		Total
	$< 60\%$	$> 60\%$	
Good	51	6	57
Insufficient	13	17	30
Negative	5	8	13
	$p < 0.0005$	$\chi^2 = 25$	

Table 5 indicates the comparison between the PCT and sperm morphology. When the percentage of anomalous forms was less than 60%, the PCT was considered good in 51 cases, insufficient in 13 and negative in five cases.

When the percentage of anomalous forms was higher than 60%, the PCT was considered good in six cases, insufficient in 17 cases and negative in eight cases. There is also a statistically significant correspondence between the PCT and sperm morphology in these values.

DISCUSSION

Our data shows that the PCT is always correlated both to sperm morphology and number of spermatozoa/ml with motility 3–4 in the first hour, and enables the *in vivo* evaluation of sperm and mucus quality. This is, therefore, an important tool during the evaluation of a sterile couple.

In our research, the PCT was negative in only four cases despite the fact that the number of spermatozoa/ml with 3–4 motility during the first hour was more than 20×10^6/ml. Regarding these four cases, the men were also subjected to immunological tests, i.e. the Mar test in seminal plasma research on the sperm-agglutinating and spermo-immobilizing antibodies in the seminal plasma and serum[8] and were positive with significant titration.

In our research, there was always a correlation between the PCT result and the quality of the sperm[9]. This means that the PCT (if accomplished when the mucus score is between 10–15) is good if the number of spermatozoa is good, and especially if the 3–4 motility of the sperm is higher than 10×10^6/ml, and the percentage of anomalous forms is lower than 60%. To underestimate and discredit the post-coital test would be easy but incorrect. Standardization is difficult; results vary from month to month and must always be repeated when unclear. However, the results of this study show that the PCT has a good correlation with semen analysis, with the number, motility and morphology of the spermatozoa themselves.

References

1. Insler, V., Bernstein, D. and Glezerman, M. (1977). Diagnosis and classification of the cervical factor of infertility. In Insler, V. and Bettendorf, G. (eds.) *The Uterine Cervix in Reproduction*, p. 253. (Stuttgart: G. Thiene Verlag)
2. Soffery, Y., Marcus, Z. H., Bukovsky, I. and Caspi, E. (1975). Immunological factors and the post-coital test in unexplained infertility. *Int. J. Fertil.*, 21, 89
3. Kovacs, G. T., Newman, G. B. and Henson, G. C. (1978). Post-coital tests: what is normal? *Br. Med. J.*, 1, 818
4. Harrison, R. F. (1980). Pregnancy successes in the infertile couple. *Int. J. Fertil.*, 25, 81
5. Moghissi, K. S. (1977). Significance and prognostic value of post-coital tests. In Insler, V. and Bettendorf, G. (eds.) *The Uterine Cervix in Reproduction*, p. 231. (Stuttgart: G. Thiene Verlag)
6. Eliasson, R. (1982). Biochemical analysis of human semen. *Int. J. Androl.*, 5, 109

7. WHO scientific group report. (1976). Agent stimulating gonodal function in the human. In Lunenfeld, B. (Chairman) WHO Consultation of the Diagnosis and Treatment of Endocrine Forms of Female Infertility. *WHO Tech. Rep. Ser. 514*
8. Hendry, W. F., Morgan, H. and Stedronska, J. (1977). The clinical significance of sperm antibodies in male subfertility. *Br. J. Urol.*, **49**, 757
9. Harrison, R. F. (1981). The diagnostic and therapeutic potential of the post-coital test. *Fertil. Steril.*, **36**, 71

Addendum to Section 2: The Biochemistry of Gonadal Function

51
Seminal plasma isoenzyme LDH-X values in extreme oligozoospermia

P. CVITKOVIĆ, M. GAVELLA, Z. PAPIĆ, Z. SINGER
and Z. ŠKRABALO

INTRODUCTION

The lactate dehydrogenase enzyme, the isoenzymes of which may be separated by electrophoresis presents one of the numerous seminal plasma constituents. Six LDH isoenzymes may be found in seminal plasma; 1–5 originate in the prostate, whereas the LDH-X isoenzyme – with an electrophoretic mobility between those of LDH 3 and LDH 4 – is associated with the presence of spermatozoa[1,2].

The LDH-X isoenzyme is a unique molecular form of LDH, first isolated in human testes and in cells of the spermatogenic line[3]. Testis homogenate studies have shown that the C gene for the C subunits of LDH-X (or LDH-C_4) becomes active in primary spermatocytes only. Correlation between LDH-X and the number of spermatozoa has been known to occur[4,5].

Conversely, to our surprise, in the investigations of extreme oligozoospermias ($> 0.1 \times 10^9/l$) two types have been observed, i.e. with low and high LDH-X[5].

It was our aim to investigate the hormonal, cytological, histological and cytogenetic testis tissue characteristics in these cases.

MATERIAL AND METHODS

A total number of 50 patients were examined, divided into two groups of 23 and 27 subjects, with high and low LDH-X respectively. Semen samples were obtained by masturbation after 4 days of sexual abstinence. LDH isoenzymes were determined by electrophoresis on 7% polyacrylamide gels, according to the Davis method[6]. The relative percentage of isoenzymes activity was estimated by means of stained gel densitometry. The high and low LDH-X percentage ranges were 10–27 and 0–4.3 respectively (0 denotes an immeasurable value on the densitometer, not necessarily indicating the absolute absence of isoenzymes).

Hormones were determined by radioimmunoassay: normal values for testosterone were 10.3–31.1 nmol/l, for FSH 2–10 U/l, and for LH 2–20 U/l, using Hypolab commercial kits. The tissue obtained by open biopsy was analysed histologically, cytologically (imprint) and for meiosis.

The normal male kariotype was confirmed in all the patients investigated by previous somatic cytogenetic examinations.

RESULTS

Table 1 shows the results obtained by hormonal analyses. The statistically significant difference between the FSH values is obvious. In subjects with low LDH-X, higher but still normal FSH levels are present.

Histological findings are presented in Table 2. Marked differences are seen with regard to the LDH-X values, revealing a tendency to stratification disorder, desquamation and obturation in cases with high LDH-X as disting-

Table 1 Relative percentage of seminal plasma LDH-X (range), plasma testosterone, FSH and LH ($\bar{x}\pm$SD) in extreme oligozoospermia

Hormones	High LDH-X (10–27)		Low LDH-X (0–4.3)
Testerone	18.2±6.4		17.9±6.2
FSH	5.5±1.3	——— $p<0.05$ ———	8.5±4.7
LH	11.5±4.3		13.9±6.5

Table 2 Histological findings

	High LDH-X	Low LDH-X
Depopulation	absent	absent
Hypospermatogenesis	absent	frequent
Diffuse fibrosis	absent	occasional
Focal fibrosis	occasional	frequent
Arrest	absent	occasional
Stratification disorder, desquamation and obturation	very frequent	rare
Spermatozoa	occasionally abundant	rare

Table 3 Cytological findings (imprint)

	High LDH-X	Low LDH-X
Spermatozoa	abundant	rare
Spermatid arrest	absent	occasional
Spermatocyte arrest	absent	rare
Spermatogonia	normal	occasionally prevailing
Sertoli's cells	normal	frequently prevailing

uished from the more frequent appearance of hypospermatogenesis and fribrosis in those with low isoenzyme values.

The results obtained by cytological analyses resembling histological findings are presented in Table 3. A marked appearance of spermatozoa has been observed in cases with higher LDH-X whereas in those with lower LDH-X spermatogonia and Sertoli's cells prevailed with some cases of arrest.

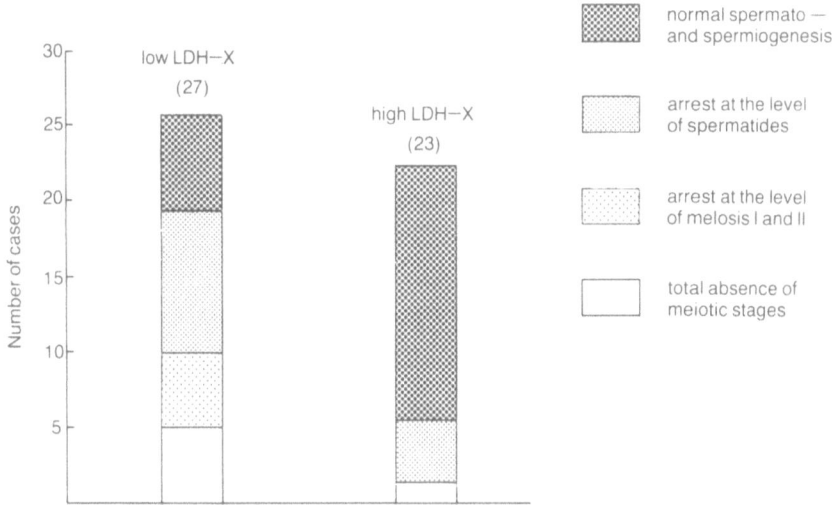

Figure 1 Cytogenetic characteristics – arrests or normal findings. All cases had normal morphology of the meiotic structures. In only one case, early division of X and Y chromosomes was observed in the metaphase I

The results of meiosis analyses are presented in Figure 1. Here the previously mentioned differences are apparent too, with the prevalence of normal findings in cases of high LDH-X.

273

DISCUSSION

Taking into account the well established correlation between the seminal plasma LDH-X values and sperm density, the results obtained in cases of extreme oligozoospermia surprised us. Obviously, the spermiogram alone proved insufficient for the assessment of the extent of the disorder in these cases. Hormonal analyses, primarily FSH, may sometimes help, but they are not sufficient for the evaluation of every particular case.

The results of our analyses indicate the existence of different sources of equally severe oligozoospermia. The results differ significantly in cases with high LDH-X compared to those with low isoenzyme. The appearance of two strictly separated types of extreme oligozoospermia thus suggests that the disorders do not occur at the same stage of spermato- and/or spermiogenesis.

CONCLUSIONS

The differences in the values of LDH-X (LDH-C_4) in the seminal plasma seem to be an adequate indicator of the total spermato- and spermiogenesis quantity and are particularly useful in the assessment of severe states such as extreme oligozoospermia. The results of this work based on histological, cytological and cytogenetic analyses of testicular tissue, and on hormonal analyses support the above statement. However, the problem of extreme oligozoospermias requires further research and obviously integrated diagnostics with a parallel analysis of the results obtained by various methods seems absolutely necessary.

References

1. Blanco, A. and Zinkham, W. H. (1963). Lactate dehydrogenase in human testes. *Science*, **139**, 601
2. Goldberg, E. (1963). Lactic and malic dehydrogenases in human spermatozoa. *Science*, **139**, 602
3. Markert, C. L. (1971). Isoenzymes and cellular differentiation. In *Advances in Biosciences 6* (Schering Symposium on intrinsic and extrinsic factors in early mammalian development) p. 511 (Oxford: Pergamon Press)
4. Rotbol, L., Hemmingsen, L. and Schmidt, V. (1969). Protein pattern and LDH isoenzymes in human seminal plasma with reference to fertility. *Clin. Chim. Acta*, **25**, 147
5. Gavella, M., Cvitković, P. and Škrabalo, Z. (1981). Seminal plasma isoenzyme LDH X in infertile men. *Andrologia*, **14**, 104
6. Davis, B.J. (1964). Disc electrophoresis II. Method and application to human serum proteins. *Ann. N.Y. Acad. Sci.*, **121**, 404

Index

AID (artificial insemination by donor)
and anejaculation, treatment, 244, 245
and counselling, 259-60
cryosperm v. fresh sperm, comparison,
    209-14
donor selection, 209-10
echosonography, and follicular growth,
    control, 205-8
and female
    pre-insemination evaluation, 218-19
    problems in, 217-21
    treatment, recommendations, 218, 219,
        220-1
follicular growth, control by
    echosonography, 205-8
pregnancy
    rate, with, 217-21
    repeat, 223-5
and problems, in female, 217-21
    treatment, 218, 219, 220-1
psychological,
    assessment of couples, 247-55
    problems of, 257-60
secrecy of, 258-9, 262-4
social roles, 261-2
success rate, 217-21
    and data interpretation problems, 217-18
AIH (artificial insemination with husband's
    semen)
indications for, 228
and post-insemination test, prognostic
    value, 227
androgen synthesis,
and human sperm coating antigen (h-SCA)
    protein, 111-15
synthesis, and prolactin, 76
    and luteinising hormone, 76
anejaculation,
aetiology, 243
definition, 243
diagnosis, 244
treatment, 244, 245-6

angiotensin converting enzyme, 69, 70
    and relaxin, effect on, 71
anosmia, and Kallman's syndrome, 135-8
antegrade ejaculation,
    drug-induced, 182, 183, 184
    and retroperitoneal lymphadenectomy,
        restoration following, 181-4, 187-9
antibiotic, and semen, bacterial
    contamination, treatment, 162, 164-5
antibody,
    antisperm, radioimmunoassay for, 123-6
    monoclonal; see monoclonal antibody
anticholinergic drug, and ejaculation,
    induction, 182
antigen,
    1113, 102, 103
    human sperm coating, analysis, 111-15
    or spermatozoa surface,
        and gel electrophoresis, 119, 120
        and cryopreservation, 117-21
antisperm antibody, radioimmunoassay for,
    123-6
artificial insemination, 203-68
    by donor; see AID
    with husband's semen; see AIH
    cervical response to, 127-30
aspermia, 181
    transport, 181
    treatment, 182-4
asthenozoospermia,
    terato, and bacteriospermia, in semen, 165
    and vitamin B_{12} level in semen, 64-7
azoospermia, and ejaculatory duct stenosis,
    191-6

bacteria, in semen, and infertility, 161-5
    antibiotic treatment, 162, 164-5
bacteriospermia, and infertility, 161-5
    antibiotic treatment, 162, 164-5
Bellak's test, and AID-demanding couples,
    psychological assessment, 248, 249-51,
    254

Bigger's, Whitten and Whittingham's
    medium, and sperm penetration test,
    27–8, 29, 30, 58, 59–60
bi-level picture processing system, and
    spermatozoa evaluation, 9–12, 23
bombesin,
    distribution, 95
    and opioid peptide, interaction, 96–7
    and pituitary gland secretion, effects on,
        95–7
bromocriptine, and ovulation, induction, 205,
    206
bromopheniramine, and ejaculation,
    induction, 182

caffeine,
    and spermatozoa motility, effect on, 38–40
        48
    and spermatozoa penetration, effect on,
        37–40
cervix, and artificial insemination, response
    to, 127–30
chinese herb medicine, and oligozoospermia,
    treatment, 155–9
clomiphene citrate, 147, 151
    and ovulation, induction, 205, 206
computer,
    and spermatozoa evaluation, 9–12, 23
    and spermatozoa velocity measurement,
        3–6
cryopreservation, of spermatozoa,
    and AID, cf. fresh sperm, 209–14
    effect on, 33–6
    non-freezing, effect on, 237–40
cyclic AMP, in sertoli cell, response to FSH
    and LH, 87

echosonography,
    and AID, follicular development, 205–8
    and follicular development, in AID, 205–8
    uses, 205
ejaculatory duct stenosis,
    causes, 191, 196
    verumontanium, transurethral resection of,
        in treatment of, 191–6
    complications, 196
ejaculatory impotence, and retroperitoneal
    lymphadenectomy, 181
    drug treatment, 182–4, 187–9
electron microscope, and sperm penetration
    studies, 51–6
emission's failure,
    drug treatment for, 182–4
    and retroperitoneal lymphadenectomy,
        treatment, 182–3

folic acid, in semen, and infertility, 63–7
FSH (follicle stimulating hormone)
    and bombesin, 96, 97
    deficiency, and Kallman's syndrome, 135–8
    release, and prolactin, 73
    and sertoli cell, response to, 85–9
    serum, and infertility, 79–84

and tamoxifen, 143, 144, 147, 148, 149,
    150, 152, 153, 154
and varicocelectomy, effect of, 177, 178

genital tract infection, chronic, diagnosis,
    91–3
gonadotrophin,
    and clomiphene citrate, 147, 151
    deficiency, isolated, 135
        and Kallman's syndrome, 135–8
    and ovulation, induction, 205, 206
    and prolactin, 76
    and tamoxifen, 147

hachimi-jiou-gan (TJ-7), and
    oligozoospermia, treatment, 155–9
heterologous therapeutic insemination; see
    AID
human sperm coating antigen (h-SCA)
    protein, 111–15
hyperprolactinaemia, and semen, cytological
    abnormality, 73–6
hypothalamus, and bombesin, 95, 97

imipramine, and ejaculation, induction, 182,
    197–9
immunology, and male reproduction, 99–130
impotence,
    ejaculatory, and retroperitoneal
        lymphadenectomy, 181
        drug treatment, 182–4, 187–9
    and testosterone undecanoate, 140–1
indirect immunoperoxidase antibody
    membrane antigen test, 118, 119
infertility,
    and autoimmunity, 123–6
    and bacteriospermia, 161–5
        antibiotic treatment, 162, 164–5
    and folic acid level in semen, 63–7
    and genital tract infection, chronic, 91–3
    psychological problems of, 257–8
    and sperm-penetration-meter test, 14–16
        possible treatment for, 16
    treatment for,
        artificial insemination, 203–8
        medical, 133–65
        surgical, 167, 200
    and vitamin B_{12} level in semen, 63–7
isolated gonadotrophin deficiency, 135
    and Kallman's syndrome, 135–8

kallikrein, and sperm motility, effect on, 48
Kallman's syndrome, 135
    treatment, 135–8
Klinefelter's syndrome, and relaxin, 70

laparoscopy, and AID, 218, 219, 220
leukocytosis, and artificial insemination,
    127–30
Leydig cell,
    and oestradiol secretion, 88–9
    and prolactin, 73

LH (luteinizing hormone)
and androgen synthesis, 76
and bombesin, 96, 97
deficiency, and Kallman's syndrome, 135–8
and hyperprolactinaemia, 74, 75, 76
and prolactin, 73, 76
and Sertoli cell, cyclic AMP response in, 87–8
and tamoxifen, 143, 144, 147, 148, 149, 150, 152, 153, 154
and varicocelectomy, effect of, 177, 178
lymphadenectomy, retroperitoneal; see retroperitoneal lymphadenectomy

Menezo B_2 medium, and sperm penetration test, 27–8, 29, 30
menotrophin, and Kallman's syndrome, 136, 137
mesterolone, and Kallman's syndrome, 136
midodrin, and ejaculation, induction, 182, 183, 184
monoclonal anti-human sperm antibody, 1113, characteristics, 101–3
and spermatozoa, membrane analysis, 105–8
mylex sheath, 244, 246

oestradiol,
secretion, and Sertoli cell, 87–9
and tamoxifen, 143, 145
oligoasthenozoospermia,
and AIH, 227
and folic acid level, in semen, 63–7
and vitamin B_{12} level, in semen, 63–7
oligospermia; see oligozoospermia,
oligozoospermia,
and chinese herb medicine, treatment, 155–9
and clomiphene citrate, 151
and FSH, 79–84
and genital duct obstruction, 79–84
and tamoxifen, treatment, 147–50, 150–54
and varicocelectomy, treatment, 175–8
and verumontanium, transurethral resection of, 191–6
and vitamin B_{12} level in semen, 64–7
ovary, follicular growth control, by echosonography, 205–8
oxedrine, and ejaculation, induction, 182

phenylpropanolamine, and ejaculation, induction, 182
penicillin, and cryopreservation, 210
pituitary gland secretion,
and bombesin, effect on, 95–7
and opioid peptide, effect on, 96–7
post-coital test,
and AIH, 227
and semen analysis, relationship between, 265–8
value of, 265
post-insemination test, and AIH, prognostic value, 227–232

pregnancy rate,
and AID, 217–21, 223–5
and spermatozoa, survival in culture medium, 233–6
and varicocoele,
following spermatic vein occlusion, 172, 173
following varicocelectomy, 175–8
Pregnyl, and Kallman's syndrome, 136
prolactin,
function in male, 73
and spermatid differentiation, 73–6
and tamoxifen, 143, 145
prostate gland,
infection, and infertility, 91–3
and prolactin, effect on, 73
and relaxin synthesis, 71
protein A, and antisperm antibody, radioimmunoassay, 123–6
puberty, delayed, and Kallman's syndrome, 135–8

relaxin,
in female, function, 69
in male semen,
function, 69–71
synthesis, 69–71
retrograde ejaculation
drug-induced, 182–4
and retroperitoneal lymphadenectomy, 181
drug treatment, 182–4, 187–9
retroperitoneal lymphadenectomy, and impotence, 181
treatment, 181–4, 187–9
Rorschach's test, and AID-demanding couples, psychological assessment, 247, 251–3, 254

scanning electron microscope, and sperm penetration studies, 51–6
semen,
analysis, and post-coital test, relationships between, 265–8
bacterial contamination, and infertility, 161–5
antibiotic treatment, 164–5
folic acid level, and infertility, 63–7
and hyperprolactaemia, effect on, 73–6
plasma protein, and human sperm coating antigen protein, analysis, 111–15
quality,
and chinese herb medicine, 155–9
and clomiphene citrate, 151
and tamoxifen, 143–6, 150–4
and testosterone undecanoate, 139–40
and varicocoele, following spermatic vein occlusion, 169–73
and variocelectomy, 176–7
vitamin B_{12} level, and infertility, 63–7
seminal vesical, and prolactin, effect on, 73
Sertoli cell,
human, in culture, 85–9
and aromatization, 88–9

Sertoli cell, human (*cont'd*)
   and FSH, response to, 87–9
   morphology, 86–7
   oestradiol secretion, 87–9
   of rat, functions, 85
   and sperm release, 75
  serum albumin, and sperm penetration
    testing, 57–60
sex therapy, and anejaculation, 244, 245–6
sperm; *see* spermatozoa
spermateleosis, and hyperprolactinaemia,
   76
spermatic vein, occlusion, and infertility,
   treatment, 169
spermatid,
  count, and infertility, 81–4
  differentiation, abnormality and
   hyperprolactinaemia, 75, 76
spermatogenesis,
  and FSH, 79–84, 88, 154
  and Kallman's syndrome, 135–8
  and Sertoli cell, FSH response, 88
  and tamoxifen, 154
  and testosterone, 154
  and varicocoele, 169
   treatment, 169–73
spermatozoa,
  abnormality, causes, 75
   and post-coital test results, comparison,
    266, 267, 268
   and tamoxifen, 143, 144, 146, 152
  antigen, 13, 102, 103
  antigenicity, and cryopreservation, effect
   on, 117–21
  antisperm antibody, radioimmunoassay,
   123–6
  ATPase activity, and prolactin, 73
  autoimmunity, 123
  capacitation, 105
  and cervical mucus penetration, bovine,
   17–20
   human, 13–16
  chromosomal analysis, 27
  coating antigen (h-SCA) protein analysis,
   111–15
  count, and AIH, prognostic value, 231–2
   and chinese herb medicine, 156–9
   and infertility, 79–84
   and tamoxifen, 147, 148, 149, 150, 152
   and varicocelectomy, 175
   and varicocoele, following spermatic
    vein occlusion, 172, 173
  cryopreservation, and antigenicity changes,
   117–21
   non-freezing, 237–40
  density, and bi-level picture processing
   system, 9–12
   and chinese herb medicine, 156, 158, 159
   and post-coital test results, comparison,
    266–7
   and tamoxifen, 143, 145
  evaluation, by bi-level picture processing
   system, 9–12

  computerised, 3–6, 9–12
  microscopic, 51–6, 57
  by sperm penetration, *see* sperm
   penetration, sperm penetration test
  by sperm velocity measurement, 3–6
  and hyperprolactinaemia, effect on, 74–6
  and leukocytosis, 127
  maturation, 105
  membrane, analysis with monoclonal
   antibodies, 105–8
  monoclonal anti-sperm antibody, 113
   characteristics, 100–3
   specificity, 107–8
  motility, and abnormality, 75
   and bi-level picture processing system,
    9–12
   and caffeine, effect on, 38–40
   and chinese herb medicine, 156, 158
   and cryopreservation, effect on, 34–6,
    237, 238, 239
   and hyperprolactinaemia, 74, 75
   laser-induced stimulation, 47–9
   and post-coital test results, comparison,
    266, 267–8
   and prolactin, 73
   and relaxin, 70, 71
   sperm immobilization test, 118–19
   and tamoxifen, 143, 144, 147, 148, 149,
    150
   and testosterone undecanote, 139, 140
   and varicocelectomy, 176–7
   and varicocoele, following spermatic
    vein occlusion, 172, 173
  penetration, *see also* sperm penetration test
   and caffeine, effect on, 37–40
   and cryopreservation, effect on, 33–6
   scanning electron microscopy studies,
    51–6
   and serum albumin, 57–60
   and spermatozoa incubation time, 57–60
   tests, *see* sperm penetration test
  survival, in culture medium, and
   pregnancy rate, 233–6
  velocity, and bi-level picture processing
   system, 9–12
   computerised measurement, 3–6
   laser-induced stimulation, 47–9
sperm immobilization test, 118–19
sperm-penetration-meter test, 13–16
sperm penetration test, and bovine culture
   medium, 17–20, 23–5
  and human culture medium, 13–16
  into zona-free hamster oocyte, 27–32
  and caffeine, effect on, 37–40
  clinical value, 41–4
  of cryopreserved spermatozoa, 33–6
  serum albumin as medium constituent,
   57–60
  and spermatozoa, pre-incubation time,
   effect on, 57–60
  and spermatozoa, velocity measurement,
   3–6
  variability, 41–4

steroidogenesis, and prolactin, effect on, 73
α-sympathomimetic drug, and induction of
  ejaculation, 182, 183, 184, 187–9

tamoxifen, and semen quality reduction,
  treatment, 143–6
  and subfertility, management, 147–50
terato-oligospermia, and bacteriospermia, in
  semen, 165
terato-zoospermia, and semen analysis,
  bacteriospermia, 161–5
testis, aromatization, 88–9
  autotransplantation, 197–200
  biopsy, and infertility, 79–84
  ductal obstruction, and infertility, 79–84
  tumor, and impotence, 181–4, 187–9
  undescended, and autotransplantation,
    197–200
testosterone, administration, problems, 139
  and clomiphene citrate, 151
  deficiency, and Kallman's syndrome, 135–8
  and human sperm coating antigen (h-SCA)
    protein, 111–15
  and hyperprolactinaemia, 74, 75, 76
  and prolactin, 73, 76

and spermatid differentiation, 76
and tamoxifen, 143, 144, 147, 148, 149,
  150, 153, 154
undecanoate, and semen quality, 139–40
  and sexual behaviour, effect on, 139,
    140–1
  and varicocelectomy, effect on, 177, 178
thyroid stimulating hormone, and bombesin,
  96, 97
transport aspermia, 181
  treatment, 182–4

urine, analysis, and infertility, 91–3

varicocelectomy, 175–8
varicocoele, and spermatogenesis, 169
  and spermatic vein occlusion, treatment,
    169–73
  and varicocelectomy, 175–8
vasography, and oligospermia, 191–6
verumontanum, transurethralresection, and
  ejaculatory duct stenosis, treatment,
    191–6
vitamin B_{12}, in semen, and infertility, 63–7